DIABETIC RETINOPATHY

By the same author :

LE DÉCOLLEMENT DE LA RÉTINE. 1968, 714 pages, 314 figures, 8 separate color plates.

Other works published by MASSON :

CORNEAL PHYSIOPATHOLOGY. 22nd International Congress of Ophthalmology. 1974, Paris, Hôtel-Dieu Symposium. 1975, 240 pages, 114 figures, 19 tables.

22nd CONCILIUM OPHTALMOLOGICUM (Paris, 1974). Acta. Papers in English, French and German. 2 volumes.
   Volume 1 — 1976, 830 pages, 291 figures (1 color illustration), 146 tables.
   Volume 2 — 1976, 1140 pages, 613 figures, 186 tables, 4 plates, 10 diagrams.

DIABETIC RETINOPATHY

by

A<small>LBERTO</small> URRETS-ZAVALIA, M.D., F.A.C.S.

Professor of Ophthalmology,
Universidad de Córdoba Medical School,
Córdoba, Argentina

117 ILLUSTRATIONS

MASSON PUBLISHING U.S.A., INC.
New York Paris Barcelona Milan
1977

MASSON Inc.   14 East 60th Street, New York
MASSON S.A.   120 Bd Saint-Germain, Paris-6ᵉ
TORAY MASSON   Balmes 151, Barcelone 8
MASSON ITALIA S.p.A.   Via Pascoli 55, Milan

Printed in France

ISBN : 0-89352-003-9
ISBN : 2-225-46310-7

CONTENTS

PREFACE

Lest someone be so inclined as to credit, or charge, me with too high an ambition, let me make clear from the start that this is not a treatise on diabetic retinopathy. It is only a brief account of my personal experience with the management of the condition. I am neither a pathologist nor a biochemist, and this small volume does not claim to be a source of information for anyone whose interests are not clinical. If I have been bound to deal with some points belonging to the laboratory sciences, this has been done diffidently and does not imply a broader range of expertise on my part.

Swift as the rhythm of medical development may appear to contemporary observers, there has not yet been any conclusive breakthrough, any watershed crossed in the case of diabetic retinopathy from the double standpoint of its pathogenesis and treatment. Progress has been made, however, and the prognosis is better today than at any time in the past. For this reason, I feel that a report of the results obtained by one worker in the treatment of a large number of patients may be of interest.

For help rendered in this book I would like to thank in particular my friend Robert C. Drews, M. D., of the Washington University School of Medicine, who was good enough to read and criticize the entire manuscript, wielding his fine editorial pen over my efforts and making many valuable suggestions; he should not be blamed for such errors as may have persisted, for in certain cases I decided to follow my own preferences. I am also indebted to my secretary, Miss Sara Morra, whose patience must have been sorely tried during these last few months. But most of all I wish to pay homage to my wife, who graciously forwent her own personal concerns in order to give support at a time when our world, and my endurance, were severely shaken.

CHAPTER 1

PREVALENCE AND IMPORT OF DIABETIC RETINOPATHY

The sheer number of publications on the epidemiology of, and the risks of blindness from, diabetic retinopathy renders collation arduous. Furthermore some of the data are approximate, contradictory and refutable. Bearing all this in mind, I have selected what seems to be the best efforts available and will present these to put our subject in perspective.

On the basis of such statistical data as were available to them, Marks *et al.* (1971) estimated that there were 3.000.000 known diabetics in the United States as of July 1, 1970. But because the onset of diabetes mellitus is typically gradual and often without obvious symptoms, or because the symptoms are ignored, an almost equal number of persons with diabetes remain undiagnosed. Accordingly, one may assume that the total number of cases at the time was approximately 5.000.000, or about 2.5% of the general population. For the world at large, the number of persons with diabetes would be about 40.000.000, even if the prevalence rate were of only 1 % (Entmacher and Marks, 1964).

Now if we note that retinopathy was present in 38 % of a representative series of diabetic patients we come to the conclusion that there must be an estimated 1.900.00 cases of diabetic retinopathy in the United States and 15.200.00 in the entire world (Bryfogle and Bradley, 1957; Bradley and Ramos, 1971).

It has long been known that the prevalence of diabetic retinopathy in any sizeable group — that is, the number of cases per unit of population on a given date — closely related ot the patients' age at the time of diagnosis, to the duration of the demonstrated retinopathy in 90 %. The scattergram to the patients' sex.

While it was believed for many years that retinopathy affected mainly older patients, it is now realized that it is alarmingly common in the young, and that it is even more frequent in patients with juvenile-onset than in those with adult-onset diabetes. Because present diabetes therapy permits an increased survival in the young, they now live long enough to develop degenerative vascular changes (Ashton, 1958). Thus, Portmann and Wiese (1954) found that retinopathy is twice as common in patients who develop diabetes before the age of 45 as in patients who become affected afterward.

That the apparent duration of diabetes is of major importance in the development of retinopathy may be seen in the major series of Waite and Beetham (1935) where the frequency of retinopathy rises from 20.5% in patients with diabetes of under 10 years duration to 58.9 % in those who have had diabetes for 15 years or longer. White and Yaskow (1948) found some degree of retinopathy in 80 % of juvenile-onset diabetics who had had the disease for 20 or more years. In a further, enlarged series of juvenile-onset patients who had had diabetes for 30 years, White (1960) demonstrated retinopathy in 90 %. The scattergram provided by Asthon summarizes the figures available up to 1958, portraying the tendency for retinopathy to increase with the duration of the disease. More recently, in a retrospective, multidisciplinary study of 73 juvenile-onset diabetic patients with 40 years or longer duration, Paz Guevara *et al.* (1974) found proliferative retinopathy in 30.1% and nonproliferative in 45.2%. Hence, it would appear that the advent of the retinal microangiopathy is almost inevitable in patients who survive.

It is difficult to determine the role of the severity of the carbohydrate disturbance, evaluated in terms of insulin requirement. Root (1955) is of the opinion that a close relationship exists between the severity of the diabetes and of the retinal involvement. In support of this he notes that the frequency of proliferative retinopathy is many times greater in the severe diabetes which begins early in life than in the mild diabetes which begins late. Even though this may be true, as an argument it is not absolutely convincing for what occurs in the growth-onset diabetic may be dependent upon the longer duration rather than upon the greater severity of the diabetic state. Indeed, the data collected by Beetham (1963) show that juvenile-onset diabetics, who are non-insulin-producers, may be better off, visually speaking, than mature diabetics, who do produce a certain amount of insulin. The remark by Root *et al.* (1959) that the diabetic aberration of the metabolism differs in patients with proliferative retinopathy in that they are generally labile, need large doses of insulin, and are difficult to control requires confirmation.

Diabetic retinopathy appears with equal frequency in women and men, but women face a somewhat increased risk of progression to blindness.

The magnitude of the scourge represented by diabetic retinopathy as a cause of blindness has been underestimated for two reasons. First, in most surveys on the causes of blindness, diabetic retinopathy is listed on a par with conditions in which the visual loss is either more easily prevented or remedied, or in which there is only a partial loss of vision from a self-limiting process. Secondly, there is the fact that, like death, blindness is susceptible of different definitions (Caird *et al.*, 1969). The notion of « legal blindness » — i.e., that of a visual acuity of less than 6/60, or a visual field of less than 20° in both eyes — has crept into all statistics and done much to confuse the issue by allowing less tragic conditions to appear statistically more impressive.

Thus, to cite but one example, in the large-scale statistics of Sorsby (1966) concerning the incidence of the various causes of blindness in England and Wales, diabetic retinopathy is recorded as a poor fifth, long after the senile macular lesions and senile cataract. This may be unquestionably correct from the standpoint of the naturalist, the nosologist, or the specialist in public sanitation and health. But not for the ophtalmic surgeon or the social worker and certainly not for the patient since (*a*) senile cataract can be operated upon successfully in the vast majority of cases, and (*b*) the loss of central vision caused by the senile maculopathies is nothing when compared to the total blindness engendered by diabetic retinopathy. This means, of course, that the burden represented by each of the diverse entities that can cause blindness depends on the extent of the visual loss entailed and that its significance changes in accordance with the therapeutic innovations brought forth by medical progress. Obviously the consequences of a disease left to its fate are one thing; those of the

same disease treated adequately are entirely different.

In this connection it is interesting to note that, although one of the calculations mentioned by Kahn and Hiller (1974) assumes that there will be a 9 % yearly increase in the number of diabetics from 1970 to the year 2000, these authors have found no evidence to support the view that the risk of blindness from diabetic retinopathy is on the rise. Accordingly, if there has actually been a substantial recent increase in the incidence — or number of new cases per unit of population per year — of diabetic retinopathy, one would speculate that treatment is now more effective in preventing blindness, since it is unlikely that the disease has started following a milder course than in previous years.

Although no one knows what the ultimate failure rate will be in those cases of diabetic retinopathy which are being treated now, of how the results achieved by the current methods of therapy will be reflected in future statistics on the causes of blindness, a point which emerges from the evidence at hand is that the two most most important conditions causing complete and irreversible loss of vision in the western world at this time are simple, open-angle glaucoma and diabetic retinopathy.

The visual prognosis in diabetes mellitus is best illustrated by the much-quoted numerical investigation of Caird and Garret (1963). These authors have found that the most important factors influencing prognosis when diabetes is first diagnosed are the presence or absence of retinopathy, the initial visual acuity, and the age at the time of diagnosis. Serial measurements of visual acuity were made over periods of up to ten years in 120 individuals with diabetic (for the most part non-proliferative) retinopathy (209 eyes) and 169 diabetics without retinopathy (309 eyes) attending the Radcliffe Infirmary Diabetic Clinic. Vision was classified into three categories: « good » if it was 6/18 or above, « impaired » if 6/24 to 6/60 inclusive, and « blind » if below 6/60. A maximum-likelihood method was used to estimate rates of exchange of category of vision in both groups of patients.

Blindness as defined developed at an estimated rate of 3 % per annum in all eyes with good vision and retinopathy, with a five-year rate of 14%; the estimated rate for eyes with good vision but without retinopathy was 0.3 % per annum. Eyes with initial visual impairment and retinopathy became blind at a much higher rate, 13 % per annum, with a five-year rate of 50 %; the control rate in eyes with impaired vision but without retinopathy was again one tenth, or 1.3 %. On the other hand, visual impairment developed in eyes with retinopathy and initially good vision at an annual rate of 7 %, the five-year rate being 34 %, whereas in the control group with good vision and no retinopathy the annual rate was 2 %. The differences between the estimated rates for eyes with and without retinopathy were all significant at the 1 % level.

Another salient factor uncovered by the same study is that the older the patient when diabetes is diagnosed the greater the chances of visual deterioration are if retinopathy is present. The trend may reflect a greater rate of progression of diabetic vascular disease in older patients; it is in keeping with the shorter duration of diabetes at the time the retinopathy sets in, and with the greater frequency of retinopathy at the time of diagnosis of diabetes among older patients. In confirmation of this, Kahn and Bradley (1975) have demonstrated that the prevalence of retinopathy is positively related to age only in diabetics with a duration of the disease of under ten years. This should mean that if youthful vasculature is protective, then ten years of diabetic disease seems to wear it out, and that if older vasculature is more vulnerable then ten years of disease is sufficient to convert more youthful retinal vasculature to equal vulnerability.

A particularly conclusive study as regards the effects of proliferative diabetic retinopathy on vision is that of Deckert et al. (1967). Fifty-one mostly juvenile-onset diabetics with proliferative retinopathy were observed for two to 18 years (average six years). The mean duration of known diabetes when proliferative retinopathy was first observed was 20.6 years. At the end of five years 10 % had died and about 50 % had become « blind » in both eyes (visual acuity 6/60 or less). These authors also noted that the visual prognosis depended upon the site and extent of the proliferative changes. Patients with localized, peripheral proliferations had a better prognosis than patients with pre- or peripapillary proliferations.

A point of interest for those more actively engaged in the treatment of diabetic retinopathy than in the management of its late complications has been raised by Patz and Berkow (1968). These investigators followed the course of 50 patients who, at the time of the first examination, had already lost vision to a level of 6/60 or less in one eye, but who still had vision of between 6/6 and 6/24 in the second eye. They found that during the first year of follow-up, vision in the second eye deteriorated to 6/60 or worse in 27 patients, or 54%. These data suggest that if the patient is to be considered for hypophysectomy or photocoagulation, the decision should be made soon after loss of vision in the first eye.

Whereas the presence of a few microaneurysms or punctate hemorrhages should not be invested with a serious prognostic significance, the presence of either proliferative retinopathy or blindness is ominous as far as life is concerned. The association of proliferative retinopathy and intercapillary glomerulosclerosis (Kimmelstiel-Wilson syndrome) is intimate. Although usually absent at the onset, hypertension, edema and persistent albuminuria almost invariably appear within months or a few years after the retinopathy. In patients under 60 the major cause of death is diabetic nephropathy with uremia. Arteriosclerotic heart disease, including coronary occlusion, is more often observed as the terminal event in the older patients (Root et al., 1959). In a short prospective study of 95 blind diabetics Patz and Berkow (1968) found that 21 % died during a 30-month period. Berkow et al. (1965) found that the average life span after the onset of blindness due to retinopathy is 5.8 years.

All this means (a) that although some diabetics can, and do, escape having retinopathy, the reason why most diabetics with retinopathy, particularly proliferative retinopathy, escape blindness is that they die prematurely, and (b) that once blindness appears life expectancy takes a turn for the worse.

CHAPTER 2

THE INDIVIDUAL FEATURES
OF DIABETIC RETINOPATHY

While most of the lesions in diabetic retinopathy can also be found in other diseases of a nondiabetic nature in which there is an impairment of the retinal blood flow but not a general metabolic disturbance, the fact remains that the different pictures seen in diabetic retinopathy are characteristic of the condition and represent a definite if protean clinical entity. Of the various elements which make up diabetic retinopathy, the primary factors are vascular, and the extravascular components are secondary. The presence and severity of the extravascular effects can nearly always be recognized with the ophthalmoscope or slit-lamp, but the detection and proper assessment of the primary vascular problems often require the use of fluorescein angiography. A broad outline of the various components of diabetic retinopathy will be given here, with an account of their histologic and pathogenetic significance. A detailed review of their clinical appearance is fully described in current textbooks and will not be repeated here. Their overall configuration and topography, their combination into several distinct pictures, and their natural course will be dealt with in the next section.

THE VASCULAR CHANGES

The basic vascular changes in diabetic retinopathy are (a) the development of areas of occlusion throughout the capillary bed, (b) the formation of microaneurysms and of anastomotic vessels, (c) the appearance of arteriolar lesions, and (d) the appearance of venous dilatation and beading. As a rule neovascularization on the retinal surface or the optic disc occurs later in the course of the disease.

The question of whether the retinal vessels differ from vessels elsewhere in the body has been answered in the affirmative. First, under normal circumstances the blood vessels of the central nervous system and retina are impermeable to the fluorescein molecule; this is not true of other blood vessels such as those of the choroid. In addition, Ashton and Cunha-Vaz (1965) and Cunha-Vaz et al. (1966) have shown that the capillaries of the retina and the brain are impermeable to tripan blue and colloidal carbon after the injection of histamine, and that the only two possible anatomical sites of such a blood-tissue barrier are the endothelial cells and the tight junctional complex which exists between them. The essential defect in many retinopathies may be a breakdown of this barrier (Ashton, 1965). This may explain why the vascular lesions of diabetic retinopathy are peculiar to the retina but are not exclusive of diabetes and occur in other vascular retinal conditions as well. True microaneurysms and new vessels do not form in organs other than the retina; but in the retina they occur not only in diabetes but also in hypertensive retinopathy, polycythemia, leukemia, the dysproteinemias, myelomatosis, pulseless disease, the aortic arch syndrome, carotid stenosis, sickle cell disease, Eale's disease, venous thrombosis, circinate retinopathy, and other diseases in which there is impairment of the retinal blood flow, hypoxia, and primary endothelial damage (Caird et al., 1969; Cunha-Vaz, 1972).

Diabetic retinal microangiopathy seems to begin in the precapillaries and capillaries, with areas of closure and focal or general dilatation (Kohner et al., 1967). At a later stage the arterioles and the veins become involved.

Foci of obliterated capillaries appear in the angiogram as sharply delineated, polygonal, dark areas of nonperfusion, situated at or near the posterior pole (Fig. 2-1). They are only 100 to 300 µ. in diameter in the early stages of diabetic retinopathy but may be much larger in the more advanced stages. They may be seen even in the mildest retinopathies. In flat retinal mounts prepared by trypsin digestion the functionless capillaries appear as empty acellular tubes of basement membrane. These capillaries lie ordinarily on the arteriolar side of the circulation and seem to be patent under the microscope. What prevents them from filling with blood in life or India ink in the injected specimen is not clear (Ashton, 1967). They arise both from occluded

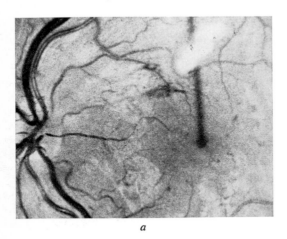
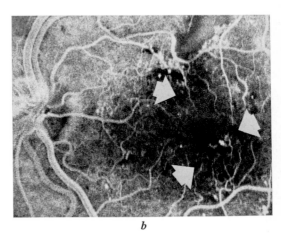

a   *b*

FIG. 2-1. — *a*) Left macular area of 24-year-old patient with early juvenile diabetic retinopathy. Note the large cotton wool spot, small scattered hemorrhages, venous engorgement, and tortuosity of some lesser vessels. *b*) A fluorescein angiogram of the same area shows in addition multiple small areas of capillary closure (arrows), microaneurysms, and marked irregularity of the arteriole which skirts the cotton wool spot.

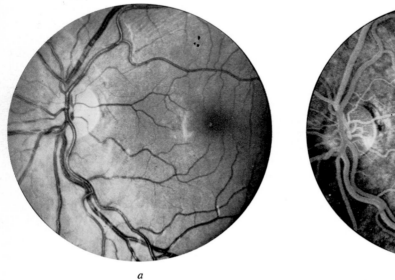
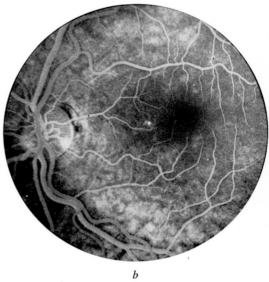

a   *b*

FIG. 2-2. — *a*) Apparently normal fundus of a 9-year-old patient with juvenile diabetes of 16 years duration. *b*) A fluorescein angiogram shows the presence of a solitary microaneurysm. This did not leak in the recirculation phase.

arterioles and from arterioles that appear to be normal. The areas of obstruction may become revascularized in time or persist indefinitely.

The adjacent capillaries, and many capillaries that are not connected with areas of visible capillary closure, show a large number of microaneurysms which vary in size from 20 to 90 μ. These are saccular and occasionally fusiform outpouchings of the capillary wall; they usually crowd together in the inner nuclear layer, along the capillaries which link the deep and superficial capillary networks (Ashton, 1958). They are the first ophtalmoscopic sign of diabetic retinopathy but may be detected by angiography in cases of latent or overt diabetes where ophthalmoscopy is negative (Fig. 2-2). They develop most commonly in the immediate vicinity of the macula or at the temporal raphe. Retinal microaneurysms have a life-cycle of their own; hypercellular and patent at

pressure. They follow and do not precede capillary damage; they develop from the pre-existing capillary bed and should not be interpreted as evidence of neovasculogenesis. Like some of the aneurysms to which they are closely associated, these varicose collateral capillaries show marked endothelial proliferation; they have been said to be particularly numerous on the venous side of the circulation. Not all areas of capillary closure possess arteriovenous collaterals (Bloodworth, 1962; Cogan and Kuwabara, 1967; Dollery, 1973). When observed by fluorescein angiography such abnormal arteriovenous communications do not seem to act as circulatory short circuits for, if anything, the transit of the dye is slower in them than in the surrounding vessels (Kohner et al., 1967). They seldom leak dye, but there are cases in which the engorged capillaries exist in such profusion and leak dye so abundantly that the whole fundus

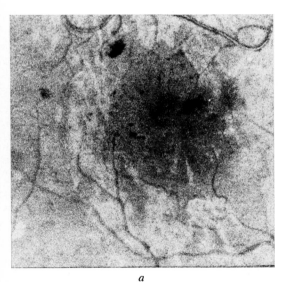
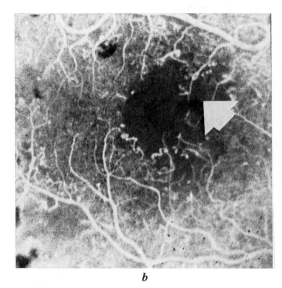

a   b

FIG. 2-3. — a) Right macular area of 21-year-old patient with early juvenile diabetic retinopathy. There are small hemorrhages and scattered red dots which could be microaneurysms or intraretinal new vessels. b) A fluorescein angiogram shows several areas of nonperfusion, one of them large (arrow), flanked and traversed by shunt vessels. Quite a few microaneurysms can now be seen.

first, they tend to fade after 12 to 24 months as they become hyalinized, suffer thrombosis, or both (Kohner and Dollery, 1970).

Traversing or flanking the areas of capillary closure are also distended and tortuous capillaries 20 to 25 μ in diameter which connect arterioles to veins and have been regarded as bypassing or shunt vessels (Fig. 2-3), dilated to accomodate a larger blood flow in response to an increased head-

seems affected by a massive intraretinal neovascularization (Fig. 2-4). These correspond to the early stages of that form af diabetic retinopathy described by Beaumont and Hollows (1972) under the name of "diffuse capillary retinopathy", which appears almost exclusively in patients under 30 years of age and follows a rapidly malignant course.

It is the contention of Davis et al. (1973) that

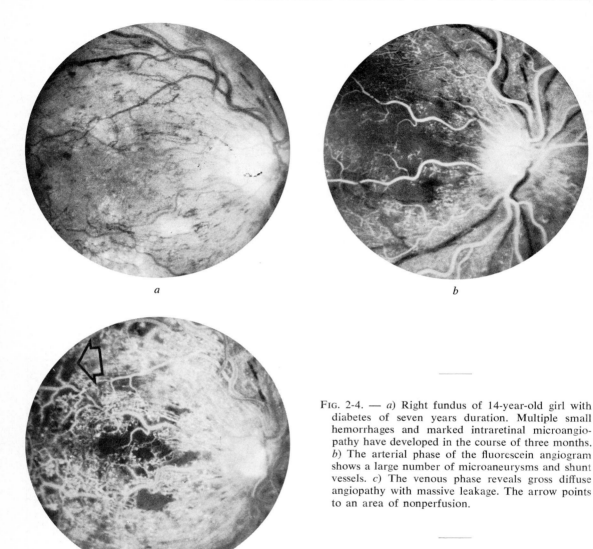

a

b

c

Fɪɢ. 2-4. — *a*) Right fundus of 14-year-old girl with diabetes of seven years duration. Multiple small hemorrhages and marked intraretinal microangiopathy have developed in the course of three months. *b*) The arterial phase of the fluorescein angiogram shows a large number of microaneurysms and shunt vessels. *c*) The venous phase reveals gross diffuse angiopathy with massive leakage. The arrow points to an area of nonperfusion.

until a better theory is advanced, the intraretinal microvascular abnormalities — i.e., both the microaneurysms and shunt vessels — are best explained as proliferations of the endothelium due to deficient blood flow.

Although not absolutely specific for diabetes, the selective destruction of the pericytes, or intramural cells, to form ghost cells, is a highly characteristic feature of diabetic retinopathy and may be of crucial pathogenetic significance (Kuwabara and Cogan, 1963). In diabetes, thickening of the basement membrane affects the entire capillary bed of the body, although perhaps not uniformly (Williamson *et al.*, 1971). When judged in flat digest specimens, the basement membrane of the retinal capillaries seems to show no appreciable thickening, or only a late thickening, except in the region of the microaneurysms and of the shunt vessels (Cogan *et al.*, 1961). But electron microscopy of the retinal capillaries (Bloodworth, 1967) shows a thickening of the basement membrane to about twice that in nondiabetic persons. Basement membrane thickening goes hand in hand with carbohydrate intolerance, and has been attributed to the possession of the diabetic genome (Siper-stein *et al.*, 1968). According to Ashton (1974) these basement membrane changes occur predo-minantly on the arterial side of the circulation, narrowing the affected vessels, and encroaching upon the lumen of the precapillary arterioles and their immediately related capillaries. This is an insidious process, which gradually interferes with metabolic exchange and with nutrition of the inner retina and of the vessel walls themselves; it results in intramural leakage and damage to the endothelial cells.

Regnault *et al.* (1973) have pointed out that the thickening of the capillary basal lamina encoun-tered in the conjunctiva of the diabetic patient varies only with the patient's age and is not related (*a*) to the duration or severity of the disease, (*b*) to the fact that the patient is or is not insulin de-pendent, or (*c*) to the degree of control achieved by medical means. In other words, it is as if this particular change were unrelated to the disturbance of the carbohydrate metabolism. But since we know that the incidence of the retinopathy is influenced by the quality of the diabetes control, and that its eventual severity does depend upon the duration of the diabetic state, we are forced to the conclu-sion that there is more to the pathogenesis of the retinopathy than a thickening of the basal mem-brane, or else that the changes in the conjunctival capillaries do not exactly mirror those in the retinal capillaries. That this is in fact the case has been demonstrated by Yodaiken and Davis (1974) who found an excellent correlation between the mean basal lamina thickness in the muscle capil-laries and severe retinopathy, but little correlation between the muscle basal lamina thickness and mild retinopathy (cf. p. 44).

The latter authors have demonstrated, moreover, that there is no significant relationship between basal membrane thickness and the capillary fra-gility for which diabetics are noted. Even those patients with the thickest basal membrane exhibit a marked increase in capillary fragility, which suggests that thick membranes provide poor support for the capillaries.

On the grounds (*a*) that an abnormal substance in the plasma of certain diabetic subjects enhances platelet aggregation, (*b*) that a correlation exists between the severity of the retinopathy and the degree of the platelet aggregation-enhancing activ-ity in the plasma, and (*c*) that platelet aggregates indeed occur in the retinal capillaries of some diabetics, it has been suggested that increased platelet aggregation favors the formation of mi-

crothrombi which lead to the development of ischemic lesions in the retina (Bloodworth and Molitor, 1965; Heath *et al.*, 1971; Regnault, 1973; Dobbie *et al.*, 1973, 1974; Lauenberger *et al.*, 1974). Since blood elements are almost never found in the lumen of nonfunctioning capillaries, one does not see how the microangiopathy of diabetes can be initiated in this manner. And yet work by Pandolfi *et al.* (1974) has shown that patients with retino-pathy have a level of the von Hillebrand antihemo-philic factor-related protein, and a antihemophilic factor activity, higher than patients without retino-pathy. The authors have suggested that since the von Hillebrand factor is involved in the mechanism of platelet adhesion and aggregation, these findings may help explain the increased platelet stickiness known to occur in diabetics, especially in those with retinal changes. The hypercoagulability of the diabetic seems to be related also to a defective fibri-nolytic system (Almér *et al.*, 1975).

While it is now evident that hypoxia plays a role in the pathogenesis of diabetic retinopathy, it is not clear whether this is ischemic or congestive in nature. In this respect it should be pointed out that some well-established facts indicate that the intraretinal blood flow is embarrassed by impaired arterial perfusion. Dollery and Kohner (1973) do not believe that the total blood flow through the diabetic retinal circulation is diminished below nor-mal. The diminished blood flow theory of the pathogenesis of diabetic retinopathy finds some support, however, in the observations by Ferrer (1974) who found that the retinal transit time is invariably increased in diabetic retinopathy, and that there exists a parallelism between the increase in the circulation time and the severity of the retinopathy, as well as a similar correlation between that increased circulation time and the augmented thickness of the capillary basal lamina as studied by muscle biopsy.

The venous changes encountered in diabetic retinopathy begin with a generalized turgescence of the main branches of the central retinal vein (Fig. 2-5). This is often found as an early sign in juvenile-onset diabetics who have no other evidence of retinopathy. As the disease progresses this venous fullness becomes more and more marked; it also loses its regularity, and a segmental dilata-tion or « beading » develops, ar does kinking, localized bulging, and reduplication. Coils or loops form and appear detached from the retinal sur-face when there is an adherence between the affected vessel and the retracted posterior hyaloid (Fig. 2-6). Occasionnally a thin channel may be seen to link the arms of an omega-shaped loop at

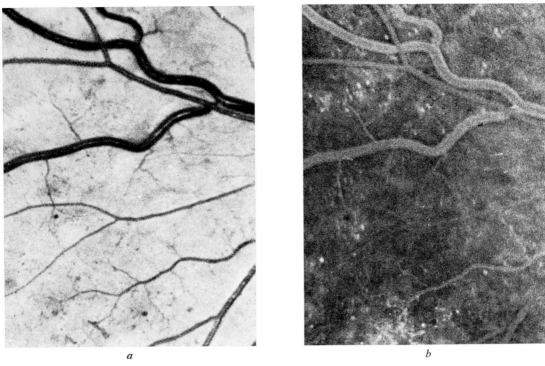

a   *b*

Fig. 2-5. — *a*) Right eye of 28-year-old patient with incipient diabetic retinopathy. There is marked dilatation of veins, blot and dot hemorrhages, and a few scattered microaneurysms. *b*) Some of the larger microaneurysms do not light up after the injection of fluorescein, but a great many others appear that were not visible, or were scarcely visible, on direct fundus examination.

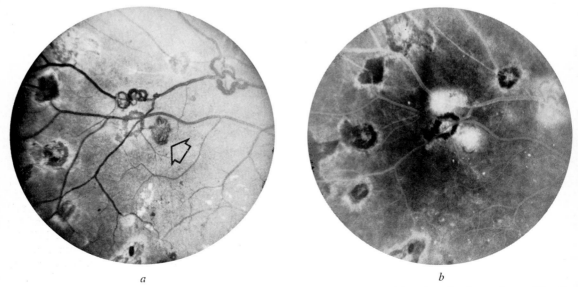

a   *b*

Fig. 2-6. — *a*) Upper temporal periphery of the right fundus of 42-year-old patient in the early proliferative phase. Note the multiple, bizarre venous coils, a rosette-shaped area of neovascularization (arrow) and several old photocoagulation scars. *b*) A fluorescein angiogram shows that dye leaks abundantly from the abnormal venous coils.

the point where they arise from the lumen of the parent vein (Doden, 1974) (Fig. 2-7).

Whereas the uniform venous dilatation seen at the outset may be reversible and is possibly only a functional alteration, the venous abnormalities encountered in the late stages of the retinopathy result from marked structural changes. The presence of severe anatomical alterations in the venous wall is revealed in the angiogram by a more or

Despite the prominent involvement of the veins encountered in almost every case of extensive diabetic retinopathy, no final answer has been given to the question of the nature and possible pathogenetic role of venous engorgement. It should be pointed out in this respect that as long as 30 years ago Cristini and Tolomelli (1947) thought that the venous dilatation seen in diabetes was primarily due to sclerosis of the precapillary arterioles, and

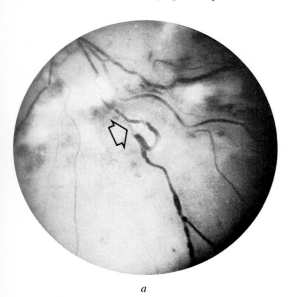 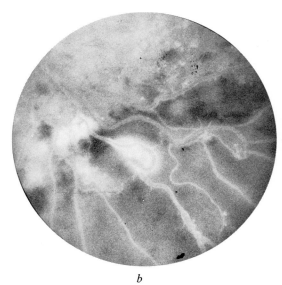

a   *b*

Fɪɢ. 2-7. — *a*) Left fundus of 68-year-old patient with diabetes of 18 years duration, and retinopathy in preproliferative stage. A large hairpin venous loop has its arms linked by a thin capillary channel (arrow). There is beading and localized bulging of the vein distally, and massive retinal edema. *b*) A late phase angiogram shows profuse leakage from the venous loop and irregular staining of the vessel wall. Note large areas of arteriolar and capillary closure.

less diffuse leakage of dye, or by a staining of the wall, seen in the recirculation stages when the lumen does not contain detectable fluorescein (Fig. 2-8). While some degree of venous distension is present in every case of diabetic retinopathy, the active proliferative form characteristically shows more advanced patterns, reminiscent of those seen in incomplete thrombosis of the central retinal vein, in macroglobulinemia, or more closely in the venous stasis retinopathy of carotid occlusion (Kearns and Hollenhorst, 1963) (Figs. 2-9 and 2-10). It should be pointed out that thrombotic obstructions of the branches of the central retinal vein are not uncommon in the diabetic patient.

The presence of gross venous anomalies is ominous; these are always coupled with vast areas of capillary closure, which sooner or later will give rise to new vessel formation.

that Ashton (1969) has failed to find any evidence of structural impediment to venous outflow in diabetic retinopathy. The view that the typical irregularities in the retinal veins should best be explained as vasoproliferation is moot, even though they are

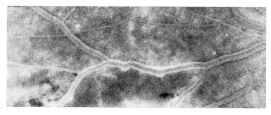

Fɪɢ. 2-8. — A fluorescein angiogram in the recirculation stages shows beading, kinking, and deep staining of venous wall. The lumen of the vein contains little detectable fluorescein.

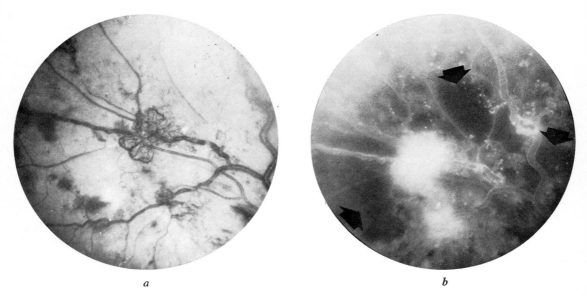

a   b

FIG. 2-9. — *a*) Upper temporal periphery of the right fundus of a 48-year-old woman with early proliferative retinopathy. Note tortuosity, distension and beading of all visible veins, as well as large tufts of epiretinal new vessels. *b*) A fluorescein angiogram shows retention of dye by the diseased vein wall, large areas of capillary closure (arrows) and profuse leakage of dye from the neovascular tufts.

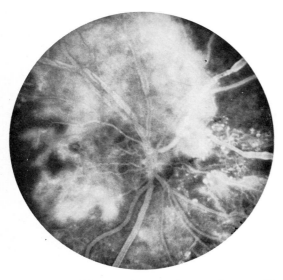

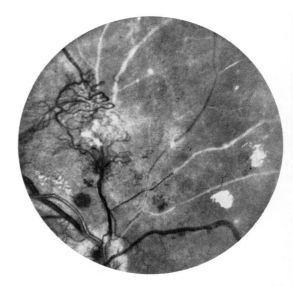

FIG. 2-10. — Venous phase angiogram from a 48-year-old patient with advanced proliferative diabetic retinopathy showing large areas of capillary nonperfusion, all manner of venous changes and massive leakage of dye from an extensive pre-papillary capillary network.

FIG. 2-11. — Upper temporal periphery of the left fundus of a 31-year-old man with early proliferative retinopathy. Note total obstruction of most arterioles of the second and third degree; also epiretinal fans of newly formed vessels.

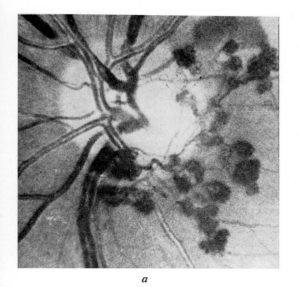

a

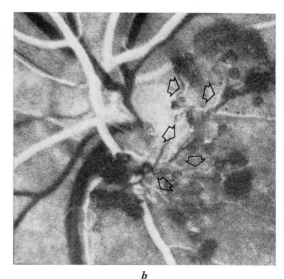

b

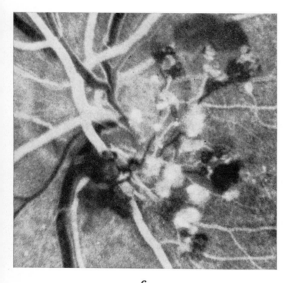

c

FIG. 2-12. — *a*) Multiple foci of berry-like, epi- and peripapillary neovascularization. *b*) An early arterial phase fluorescein angiogram shows feeding channels to most of the neovascular coils (arrows). *c*) In the early venous phase the arterial supply to the new vessel system can no longer be identified.

often the harbinger of impending vasoproliferation (Davis *et al.*, 1973).

The arteriolar changes found in the retina by Ashton (1952) consist mainly in a hyaline degeneration which may be as severe as that which occurs elsewhere in the vascular system. This hyalinization leads to a gradual narrowing of the terminal arterioles and precapillaries which, apart from a diffuse circulatory insufficiency involving the whole retina, has also been known to cause focal ischemia and infarction. The distal portions of the larger arterioles and the smaller arterioles appear oph-

thalmoscopically as if affected by involutionary sclerosis: they are pale and straight, and show a pipe-stem sheathing or even (when fibrosis of the media and the intima is very advanced) a total obliteration (Fig. 2-11). The affected vessels lie in the mid-periphery of the fundus or are adjacent to areas of capillary closure at the posterior pole, where they have protrusions or stumps which probably represent pruned off side branches. In the angiogram the occluded arterioles may not fill with fluorescein. In those still patent the diseased wall becomes impregnated with the dye.

In some cases of diabetic retinopathy arteriolar obliteration is widespread, involving both small and large order arterioles, and becomes the predominant feature of the disease (Bresnick *et al.*, 1975). It advances rapidly and is associated with extensive areas of capillary nonperfusion and with marked venous dilatation. Ischemic maculopathy causes profound loss of vision. There is optic disc pallor and neovascularization, and a high incidence of rubeosis iridis with neovascular glaucoma. Neovascularization represents the initial proliferative change. The clinical occurrence, appearance and natural course of this most serious vascular alteration, and of the accompanying fibrotic framework, will be discussed in the next chapter. For the time being let us say that the new vessels are thin-walled and leak fluorescein from the early arteriovenous phase. Microaneurysms are never seen on new vessels. Flow through them is ordinarily sluggish. They originate in an endothelial budding process which has been said to prevail in the venous side of the circulation. The obvious fact is, however, that in the angiogram they start to fill during the early arterial phase and seem to be related more intimately to the arteriolar tree than to the venous tree. There is also the fact that many new vessel systems of either the fan-like, the berry-like or the arborizing variety are connected to an arterial feeding channel which can be detected by fluorescein angiography (Kohner *et al.*, 1967) (Fig. 2-12). As will be seen later, one of the most effective schemes for photocoagulation treatment demands that this feeding vessel be identified and destroyed. The new vessels are permeable to plasma proteins which pass into the vitreous, alter its colloidal state, and help produce a posterior vitreous detachment even before a hemorrhage occurs.

The stimulus which causes neovascularization — the factor X of Wise (1956) — is as yet unknown; it seems to be formed by an inadequately perfused retina. It has been suggested, however, that hypoxia may not be the correct explanation for the formation of new vessel systems because these vessels sometimes arise in areas where the circulation is comparatively normal and not from areas of widespread destruction, where tissue hypoxia must be more severe (Kohner *et al.*, 1967). If the retina is in its normal position against the choroid — which Cogan and Kuwabara (1967) showed to be relatively immune to specific diabetic angiopathy — its outer layers will be normally oxygenated by the choriocapillaris. Vasoproliferation will therefore be produced only in the inner layers and overflow into the vitreous.

As may be seen from the foregoing, our understanding of the disease process involved in diabetic retinopathy is based on a number of loosely connected and even contradictory data. Our only hope is that sometime, somehow, other additional clues fall into place until the whole picture emerges.

THE EXTRAVASCULAR COMPONENTS
OF DIABETIC RETINOPATHY

Lesions of a hemorrhagic, exudative, or necrotic character appear in the tissues surrounding the changes in the retinal vasculature that have just been described. There are first, of course, the retinal and retro- or intravitreal hemorrhages; secondly, the edema of the central retina and the hard or waxy exudates; and thirdly the cotton-wool patches.

The extravasation of whole blood is of prime importance. The early hemorrhages in diabetic retinopathy are the typically rounded dot and blot red spots (Fig. 2-5); they occur deep in the retinal structures, especially in the inner nuclear and outer plexiform layers (Henkind, 1973). The flame-shaped hemorrhages often encountered in older patients lie superficially in the nerve fiber layer and result from arterial hypertension rather than from the diabetic state (Fig. 2-13). Later the hemorrhages may be of any size and shape, and affect all the retinal layers (Fig. 2-14); they may break through the internal limiting membrane and enter the vitreous cavity. The irruption of red blood cells out of the vascular lumen reveals that a break in the continuity of the vascular wall has taken place, since the red blood cells are incapable of diapedesis.

As noted by Davis (1967), intraretinal edema is not rare, as stated generally, but is rather one of the commonest components of diabetic retinopathy. It involves the macular region predominantly and can be overlooked by indirect and even by direct ophthalmoscopy. The thickening of the retina to which it gives rise can be assessed only by means of the slit-lamp and a flat contact lens, or in stereoscopic fundus photographs. Reliable information on the severity of macular involvement can be gained from late phase angiograms, which show the extent and degree of fluorescein leakage (Fig. 2-15). The natural course of the edema is toward the formation of pockets of fluid located in the outer plexiform layer with subsequent cystoid degeneration.

the dye; (c) the lipid clears up after destruction of the abnormal vessels by photocoagulation; (d) it also clears up when the patients are placed on a low-fat diet; and (e) visual acuity may improve after the deposits in the macular area are absorbed (Maumenee, 1968). Nevertheless, the possibility that a small part of the material in question represents a breakdown product of degenerated neural cells cannot be dismissed altogether (Bloodworth, 1962 and 1963).

The cotton-wool spots or soft exudates appear as isolated, fluffy white patches (Figs. 2-1 and 2-

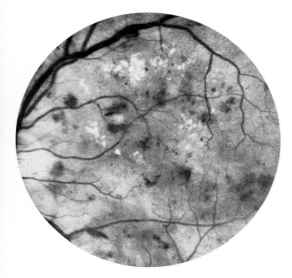

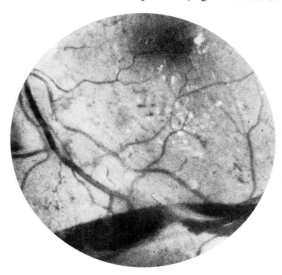

FIG. 2-13. — Left fundus of a moderately hypertensive patient showing multiple blot hemorrhages interspersed with small flamed-shaped hemorrhages and a few discrete hard exudates.

FIG. 2-14. — A typical boat-shaped (in this case bilocular) preretinal hemorrhage in its usual location under the disc and macula.

As plasma leaks from the damaged vessels, fluid is absorbed by the surrounding intact capillaries more rapidly than are the blood constituents with large molecules. A selective accumulation of lipids ensues, which leads to the formation of the deposits known as hard exudates (Fig. 2-16). Like the edema itself, these appear at the posterior pole and lie predominantly in the outer plexiform layer. They are composed of lipoproteins, glycoproteins and phospholipids, with an admixture of neutral fats (Yanko *et al.*, 1974). At the present time there does not seem to be any doubt as to the source of the material in the hard exudates. The arguments in favor of the concept that it is derived from the blood are many: (a) the deposits appear around or at the margin of the vascular lesions; (b) fluorescein angiography reveals that the wall of the defective vessels or microaneurysms is permeable to

17). They are infarcts due to acute arteriolar obstruction and correspond to areas of localized swelling and axon disruption located in the nerve fiber layer of the retina (Ashton, 1970). They develop at the posterior pole, predominantly in the area of distribution of the radial peripapillary precapillaries. Their turnover rate is slower than in hypertension, some lesions persisting for over a year without apparent change. Clearance probably depends upon the speed of revascularization and entry of microphages (Dollery, 1973). The minute arterioles which end in the cotton wool spots are extremely narrowed or occluded and they frequently leak fluorescein (Dollery and Kohner, 1973). Although the occurrence of an occasional soft exudate is common in diabetic retinopathy, even in the absence of concomitant hypertension, the simultaneous appearance of a number of them constitutes an unfavorable sign. Like the development of marked beading of the veins, which acquire a string-of-sausages appearance and a dark plum color, it bodes ill for the patient in that it usually is the forerunner of an upsurge in hemorrhagic activity, or of an imminent or renewed tendency to new vessel formation.

Among the nonretinal ocular disorders which appear as a consequence of the initial vascular changes in diabetic retinopathy one should lay stress upon those affecting the vitreous body. Although secondary in the main to the lesions in the retina itself, the altered conditions in the vitreous can lead in turn, as we shall see, to an impairment of the very same lesions that triggered their appearance.

Bleeding into the vitreous from any source — microaneurysm, distended vein, new formed vascular tuft — creates a disturbance in its colloidal state. The presence of hemoglobin causes a depolymerization of the hyaluronic acid, and fibrin a breakdown of the collagen framework. But even if a hemorrhage has never occured, leakage of protein from the new vessels on the optic nerve-

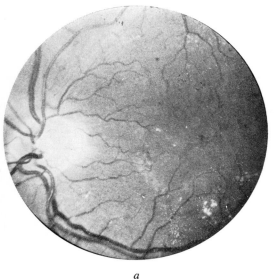

a

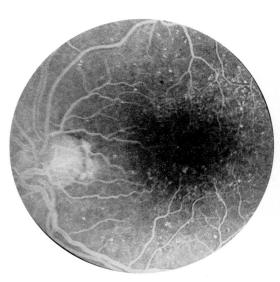

b

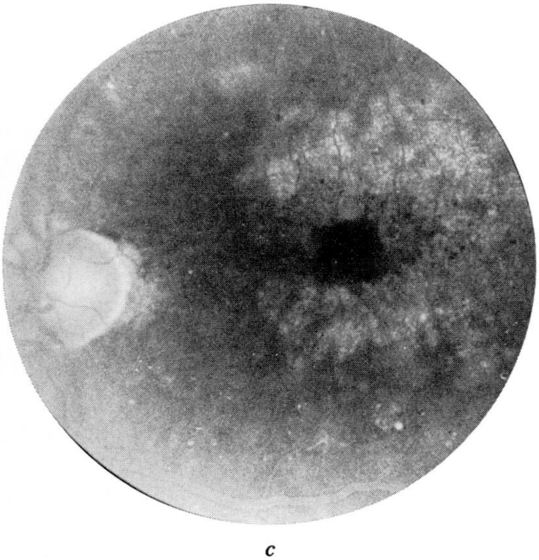

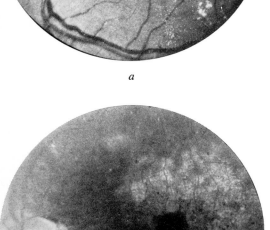

c

FIG. 2-15. — *a*) Left fundus of 59-year-old man with diabetes of ten years duration. Only a few punctate hemorrhages or microaneurysms and a few tiny fatty exudates are seen. *b*) An early venous phase fluorescein angiogram shows a large number of microaneurysms around the capillary-free zone at the fovea and temporal to it. *c*) A late phase angiogram shows deep intraretinal leakage of dye; the fovea is threatened but not yet involved by the disease process. The vessels no longer contain any visible dye.

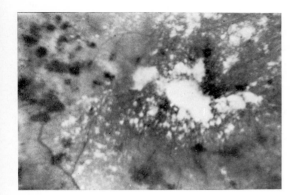

FIG. 2-16. — Right fundus of 54-year-old woman suffering from diabetic maculopathy. Note multiple, partly confluent hard exudates, scattered micro-aneurysms, and rather large blot hemorrhages. On examination with the slit-lamp and a flat contact lens, a marked retinal edema was found.

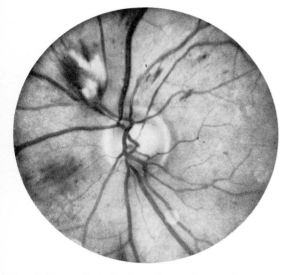

FIG. 2-17. — Left fundus of a patient with marked hypertension (220/100 mm Hg), and diabetes of 11 years duration. Note the large soft exudate surrounded by flame-shaped hemorrhages; other dot, blot, and flame-shaped smaller hemorrhages are scattered throughout the fundus.

head or the retinal surface has a similar effect, which may be recognized from the vitreous haze that is seen to develop. As the vitreous gel suffers it contracts and detaches posteriorly, and a thickening and loss of transparency of the posterior hyaloid occurs.

Depending on the mechanism of the transfer of fluid from the vitreal into the retrovitreal space,

Eisner (1973) distinguishes between a rhegmatogenous (degenerative) and an arrhegmatogenous (secondary to a pathologic condition of the adjoining tissues) type of vitreous detachment (Fig. 2-18). In the first type, which is a result of ageing or of high myopia, there is a hole in the posterior hyaloid membrane through which the destroyed liquified vitreous can pass into the newly formed retrovitreal space. In the second type, which is that seen in diabetic retinopathy, fluid transfer is effected through the intact hyaloid membrane. Consequently, the posterior vitreous detachment encountered in the diabetic patient with retinopathy differs in several respects from that seen in old people and in myopes:

1. Its occurrence is not necessarily preceded by syneresis, i.e., by fibrillar and lacunar degeneration; it is not associated with the sudden collapse seen in the purely degenerative type of vitreous detachment.

2. It develops gradually rather than abruptly, and is not attended by the usual appearance of floaters or shower of minute opacities.

3. It does not affect simultaneously, or completely, the entire area of contact between the posterior hyaloid and the internal limiting membrane, so that some adherences persist in addition to the normal anchorage of the vitreous base to the pars plana and peripheral retina.

4. Tearing of the retina and rhegmatogenous retinal separation occur oftentimes in the case of the degenerative type of vitreous detachment; conversely, the formation of retinal folds or a traction retinal detachment is more characteristic of the secondary type.

5. In contrast to the highly mobile posterior detachments found in the absence of any major disease, the posterior vitreous separation in diabetic retinopathy is more rigid and may progress to the point where the shrunken gel stretches across the eye as a frontally oriented membrane.

The effect of this retraction upon the normal or new-formed vessels attached to the posterior vitreous face and upon the inner retinal layers from which these proceed is catastrophic. The fundus changes brought about by vitreous contraction include : avulsion of isolated retinal vessels and elevation of fibrovascular tissue; retrohyaloid and intravitreal bleeding; traction retinoschisis and detachment of the retina; and plicature of the retina (Bresnick *et al.,* 1975).

In exceptional cases, a unilateral or bilateral

optic neuritis may occur in uncontrolled diabetes. This is usually of little severity and leaves only some atrophy of the disc with a moderate decrease in visual acuity and a concentric field defect. It has been attributed to toxic metabolic changes or more plausibly to a disorder in the capillary network of the optic nervehead (Yanko *et al.*, 1972).

A more severe form, associated with both diabetes mellitus and diabetes insipidus, occurs mostly in the young, is linked to a special genetic factor, and may be due to an adhesive arachnoiditis at the level of the optic chiasm (Damaske *et al.*, 1975) (Fig. 2-19).

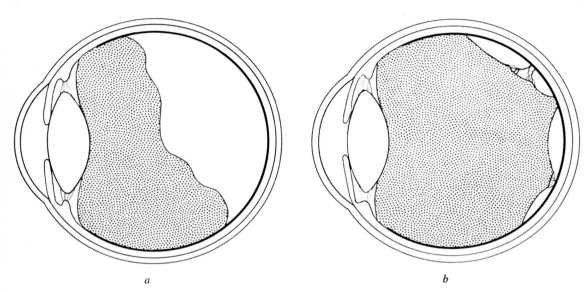

a   *b*

Fig. 2-18. — *a*) Schematic representation of the degenerative or rhegmatogenous type of posterior vitreous detachment which is the result of ageing or of high myopia. The posterior hyaloid membrane is regularly convex, mobile, and shows no adherence to the retinal surface; the main mass of the vitreous substance lies on the lower part of the retina. *b*) Arrhegmatogenous or secondary type of vitreous detachment as seen in diabetic retinopathy, where the posterior hyaloid is taut between pre-existing adherences to the retinal surface, and the shrunken vitreous substance appears rigid.

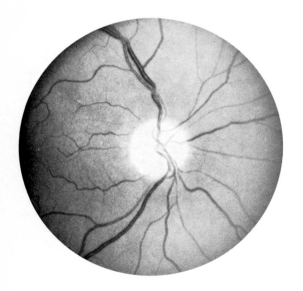

Fig. 2-19. — Pronounced optic atrophy as seen in a 28-year-old man with diabetes of 21 years known duration. Corrected visual acuity was 5/50 in both eyes. Note the absence of diabetic retinopathy. Fluorescein fundus angiography was noncontributory.

CHAPTER 3

MAJOR CLINICAL TYPES AND NATURAL COURSE
OF DIABETIC RETINOPATHY

A suitable classification of diabetic retinopathy should include the possibility of describing qualitatively and quantitatively the various clinical pictures at initial and subsequent examinations, of recording by fundus photography and fluorescein angiography the lesions existing in predetermined areas, and of establishing the natural course of the malady.

While the so-called O'Hare classification (cf. Goldberg and Fine, 1968), which is simple and easy to keep in mind, proved most useful in the case of proliferative retinopathy, the method devised by Oakley et al. (1967) afforded a better means of assessing the severity of the condition, inasmuch as it (a) requires a comparison of its various components with a set of standard photographs, and (b) gives a numerical grade to the same, allowing for statistical analysis. Better still than the latter, usually referred to as the Hammersmith classification, and than several others such as those of Lee et al. (1966) and of Okun et Cibis (1966), which were based on a series of diagrams and suffered from lack of universal acceptance, is the Airlie House classification, which combines the advantages of the above but manages to avoid their major drawbacks (Davis et al., 1968). Based on 15 pairs of fundus stereographs and to a lesser degree on written descriptions, it should be utilized in every prospective study aimed at evaluating objectively the effectiveness of a therapeutic approach or the spontaneous changes occurring in the individual case.

However, for discussing the manner in which diabetic retinopathy can be treated, what is needed is not so much an *analytic* method of gauging the severity of the individual case at appropriate intervals as a less elaborate system serving to identify the different forms of the disease. Though of great nosological merit, the classifications of Ballantyne and Michaelson (1947), Scott (1951, 1953) and Alaerts and Slosse (1957) do not lend themselves to this end.

Being purely descriptive and *synthetic* in nature, the following arrangement does not imply that the categories listed should be regarded as stages which appear necessarily in a regular sequence. Also, on account of the sheer weight of their diverseness, the writer has had to restrict himself to the more frequent and important ones. But even if not entirely satisfactory in many respects, the grouping which has been chosen seems to be apposite in that it is conducive to an orderly presentation and provides us with a frame of reference within which any remedial steps may be discussed adequately. The division of diabetic retinopathy into the two conventional types designated as simple, or background, and proliferative has of course been retained. A further separation of each type into a number of subtypes was considered necessary.

SIMPLE RETINOPATHY

Simple, background or nonproliferative retinopathy should be regarded as a direct reflection of the diabetic microangiopathy occurring in the peculiar anatomic structures of the eye. Pathologically its hallmark lies in a thickening of the capillary basement membrane and in the appearance of acellular capillaries with death of the pericytes. Ophthalmoscopically, it is signified by the development of microaneurysms and distended intraretinal vessels. As a rule it assumes either a predominantly hemorrhagic character or an equally predominantly exudative character although it often combines the features of both (Duke-Elder and Dobree, 1967).

I. — HEMORRHAGIC NONPROLIFERATIVE RETINOPATHY

In its hemorrhagic form, simple retinopathy is usually seen in younger diabetics who have developed the disease in the early years of life, although this is not by any means necessarily so (Figs. 3-1

edges, the so-called soft exudates or cytoid bodies, are foci of ischemia resulting from an obstruction of the adjacent arterioles by fibrinoid necrosis.

Retinal dot, linear, and flame-shaped hemorrhages appear early. Scattered all over the retro-equatorial fundus but mostly in the region enclosed by the main vascular arcades, they are initially small but become subsequently larger and confluent, and may break through the internal limiting membrane into the preretinal space. Their starting-point is not clear: although frequently derived from the aneurysms, as assumed originally by MacKenzie (1877) and Nettleship (1888), they

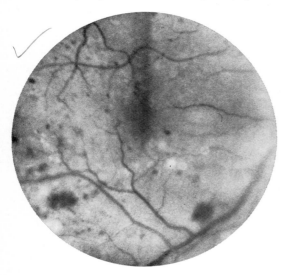

FIG. 3-1. — Early case of purely hemorrhagic diabetic retinopathy in a 24-year-old man.

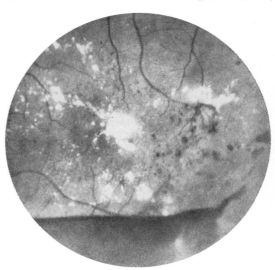

FIG. 3-2. — Predominantly hemorrhagic form of diabetic retinopathy in 56-year-old patient. There are a number of dot and blot hemorrhages lateral to the macula and a navicular hemorrhage inferiorly. Also present are multiple small fatty exudates with early plaque formation.

and 3-2). In those cases which are doomed to follow a malignant course it amounts to what should be regarded as the preproliferative stage (Fig. 3-3).

It begins as a uniform dilatation and tortuosity of the larger veins and their primary branches. As the turgescence increases, variations in caliber occur, until a marked irregularity develops in the form of multiple constrictions with beading or sausaging that may be associated with other abnormalities. Arteriovenous shunt vessels, which link an artery directly to a vein and are usually larger in diameter than normal capillaries, surround or cross the zones of nonperfusion revealed by angiography. At a somewhat later stage, damage to the small and medium-sized arteries is common at a distance from the posterior pole.

Faint, whitish, cotton-wool spots with indistinct

may have their origin in some of the affected veins, the walls of which are fragile as a result of hypoxia.

II. — EXUDATIVE NONPROLIFERATIVE RETINOPATHY

In its exudative form, background diabetic retinopathy is usally seen in the maturity-onset patient. The prevailing microangiopathy is most easily identified ophthalmoscopically as clusters of microaneurysms, some varicose capillaries, shunt vessels and punctate hemorrhages arranged in a few foci

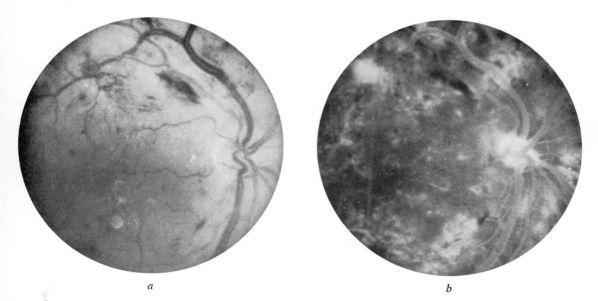

a   *b*

Fɪɢ. 3-3. — *a*) Right fundus of 54-year-old woman with diabetes of 11 years duration. Note irregular engorgement of retinal veins, some scattered microaneurysms, and numerous blot and flame-shaped hemorrhages; there are also a few wispy, isolated epiretinal new vessels: the patient is in an early proliferative stage. A marked edema of the macula could be seen on biomicroscopic examination. Corrected visual acuity: 5/40. *b*) In the venous phase fluorescein angiogram massive leakage appears which involved the entire posterior pole, including the macula.

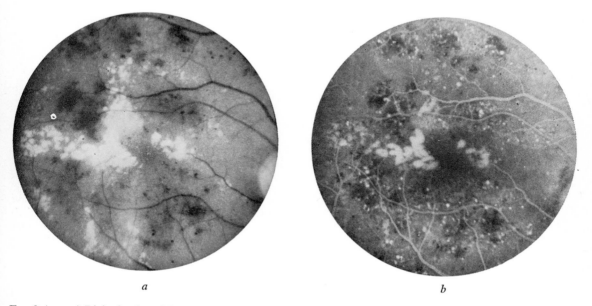

a   *b*

Fɪɢ. 3-4. — *a*) Right fundus of 37-year-old man suffering from typical exudative maculopathy. Multiple medium-sized, partly confluent, hard, waxy deposits occupy the macula, surrounding the fovea. There are numerous scattered microaneurysms and large blot hemorrhages. Corrected vision was 5/10. *b*) Venous phase fluorescein angiogram showing innumerable microaneurysms.

which lie at the posterior pole, often lateral to the macula (Fig. 3-4). Eventually, leakage from the damaged vessels will give rise to an edema of the macula where the retina may be swollen to four or five times its normal thickness. Although largely reversible at first, this edema may lead to microcystoid degeneration, macrocystic degeneration, and even to the formation of a macular hole. Hard, waxy deposits develop in the macula and its vicinity as a result of the extravasation of plasma. They appear as small scattered flecks of lipoid material or as conglomerates of variable size, from rings covering a fraction of a disc area to wreath-like aggregations several disc diameters across; they may also merge into large plaques which encroach on the fovea (King *et al.,* 1963; Dobree, 1970) (Figs. 3-5 and 3-6). As previously noted, they are due to leakage from the damaged capillaries and result in neuronal destruction.

Most of these cases have minimal extramacular manifestations of diabetic retinopathy, with little or no venous changes, no significant hemorrhagic activity and few if any proliferative signs. The high incidence of this sort of pathology in the

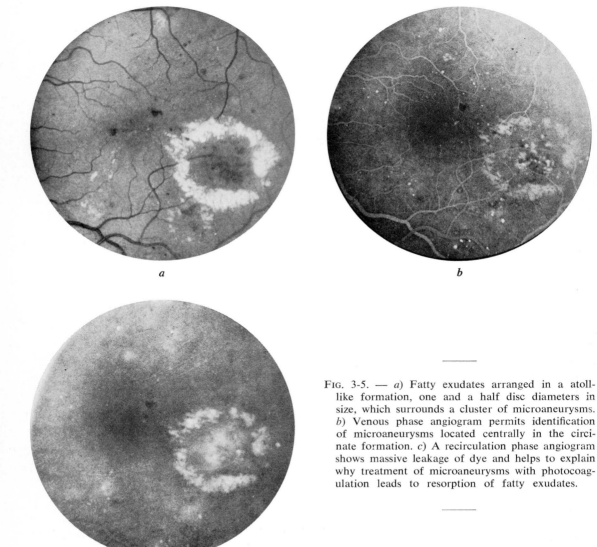

a

b

c

Fig. 3-5. — *a)* Fatty exudates arranged in a atoll-like formation, one and a half disc diameters in size, which surrounds a cluster of microaneurysms. *b)* Venous phase angiogram permits identification of microaneurysms located centrally in the circinate formation. *c)* A recirculation phase angiogram shows massive leakage of dye and helps to explain why treatment of microaneurysms with photocoagulation leads to resorption of fatty exudates.

older age group, in which it acts as the sole vision-threatening expression of the disease, seems dependent upon the premature ageing of the diabetic's vasculature and the more general fact that the breakdown of the small blood channels in response to hemodynamic stress is fostered by the presence of atherosclerotic changes.

Serial fluorescein angiography in background retinopathy of both the hemorrhagic and exudative forms reveals that not all the bright red spots seen on direct examination and color photographs fill or stain with the dye. In many cases, large aneurysms displayed prominently in the photographs corresponding to the arterial or early venous phase show no significant diffusion into the surrounding tissues. In others, intraretinal microvascular abnormalities that are only dimly visualized in the control pictures show heavy leakage in the late phases of the dye transit. The value of fundus angiography lies also in the demonstration of areas of avascularity or capillary closure, which appear as irregular dark patches surrounded by truncated vessels and multiple microaneurysms.

Characteristically, in the hemorrhagic form, some segments of the distended and tortuous venules and even arterioles become impregnated so that their wall continues to fluoresce after the lumen no longer contains detectable dye. Both the irregularities in caliber and the prolonged retention of the dye in the wall of the affected vessels are embodied in the notion of a diffuse angiopathy (Balodimos *et al.,* 1968). In the exudative form

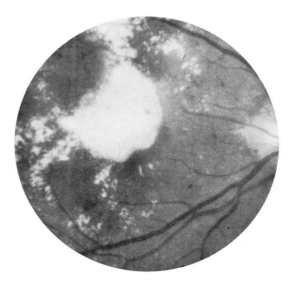

FIG. 3-6. — A purely exudative type of diabetic retinopathy showing multiple hard deposits with advanced plaque formation. Only a few scattered microaneurysms can be seen and no hemorrhages are present.

with macular edema, fluorescein fundus photography will enable the observer to distinguish between cases with only localized leakage and cases with diffuse leakage at the posterior pole (Figs. 3-7, 3-8 and 3-9).

PROLIFERATIVE RETINOPATHY

Proliferative retinopathy is marked by the development of gliovascular tissue on the surface of the retina, on the nervehead, and into the vitreous. As a cause of recurring hemorrhages it may be superimposed on a simple retinopathy that has remained stationary or only slowly deteriorated for years in the maturity-onset patient (Fig. 3-10). It may also occur in eyes that have had little or no previous changes, notably in the labile, insulin dependent, growth-onset patient (Figs. 3-11 and 3-12). The first situation emanates from the natural progression of the disease; it should be regarded as an expression of the gradual impairment of circulatory conditions in the retina or, more rarely, as an organizational process, in the

form of fibrous membranes which develop after repeated bleeding into the vitreous (cf. p. 30). The second situation, in which the vasoproliferative changes occur for the most part without history or evidence of vitreous hemorrhage, represents a special type of diabetic manifestation rather than a terminal stage, or at least a distinct process within the wider concept of diabetic retinopathy (Fisher, 1963; Cogan, 1964).

Though one may attempt to isolate the individual phases of proliferative retinopathy for purely descriptive purposes, it must be kept in mind that one is always dealing with a conjugation of variants. Consequently, every single case in this category will be apt to exhibit some of the

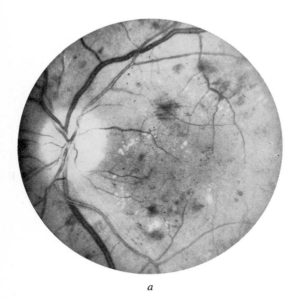

a

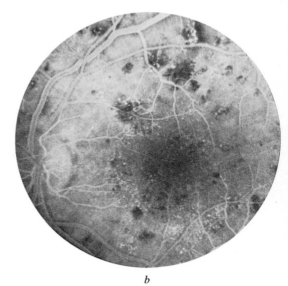

b

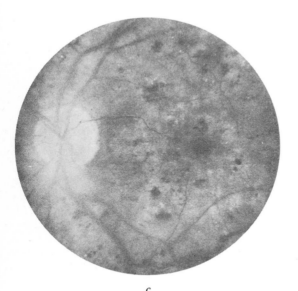

c

Fɪɢ. 3-7. — *a*) A predominantly hemorrhagic form of nonproliferative retinopathy in the left eye of 48-year-old man. Note microaneurysms; dot, blot, and flame-shaped hemorrhages; and small scattered hard exudates. Visual acuity: 5/10. *b*) Venous phase fluorescein angiogram showing many more microaneurysms than were apparent on direct examination. *c*) Recirculation phase angiogram showing barely discernible leakage of dye deep in the retinal structures.

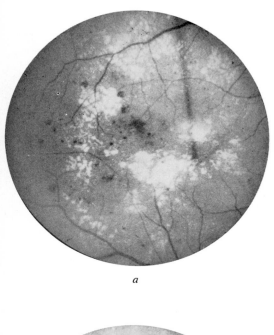

a

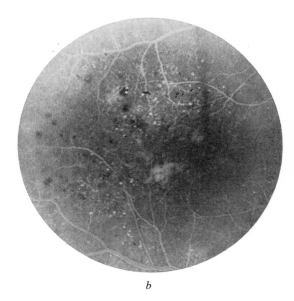

b

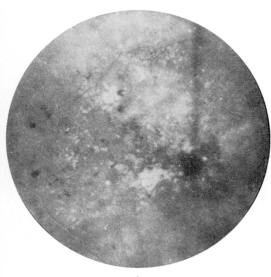

c

FIG. 3-8. — *a*) Exudative diabetic retinopathy in 68-year-old woman whose other eye suffered from a dense intravitreal hemorrhage of three years duration. *b*) A venous phase fluorescein angiogram shows multiple microaneurysms but no gross vascular abnormalities. *c*) In the recirculation phase angiogram there is moderately profuse leakage of dye in the region between the temporal vascular arcades.

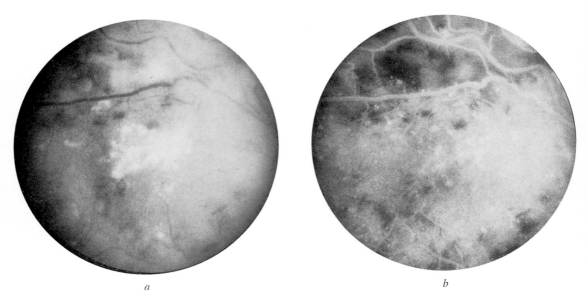

a   *b*

FIG. 3-9. — *a*) Advanced form of exudative retinopathy with marked venous changes, diffuse retinal edema and partly confluent hard deposits in the upper macular area; a few blot hemorrhages are present. *b*) An early venous fluorescein angiogram shows massive leakage of dye which does not spare the fovea.

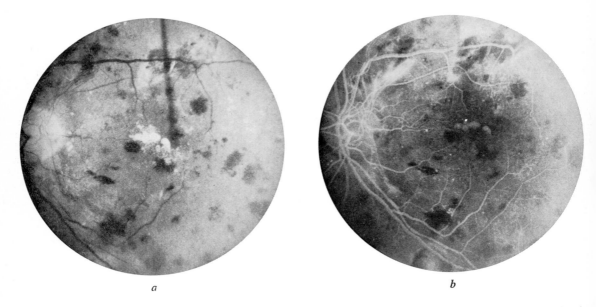

a   *b*

FIG. 3-10. — *a*) Early proliferative retinopathy which appeared as a complication of a simple retinopathy in 56-year-old man with diabetes of 24 years duration. Note thin neovascular tufts and isolated, tendril-like bare vessels which arise from the disc and advance well into the papillomacular area. *b*) A venous fluorescein angiogram shows leakage from neovascular formations.

point. The point is that, apart from an unforeseen — and ordinarily fleeting — turn for the better, only a deterioration in the state of the fundus can be anticipated, and that, in general, such periods of inactivity as are usually observed belong to the final stages of the condition, when they can hardly be regarded as an amelioration for at this point in time vision has been irretrievably lost.

From what has been said the conclusion arises that blindness — at least legal blindness, or vision under the 6/60 level — comes as an upshot of:

(*a*) loss of macular function,

(*b*) repeated or copious intraocular hemorrhages which obscure the red reflex of the fundus,

(*c*) massive fibrous proliferation which overshadows the posterior pole, or

(*d*) retinal detachment.

Blindness may also result from neovascular glaucoma, which may develop swiftly in eyes that present only moderate retinal changes (not necessarily even proliferative) and which may benefit transiently from cyclocryotherapy.

CHAPTER 4

METHODS OF CLINICAL EXAMINATION

The examination of a person suffering from overt diabetic retinopathy, or even a person in whom the presence of latent retinopathy is suspected, should include a detailed ophthalmic history; general medical history; accurate refraction and visual acuity test; tonometry; biomicroscopy of the anterior segment and lens before and after pupillary dilatation; binocular indirect ophthalmoscopy; direct ophthalmoscopy; and serial fundus photography following the intravenous injection of sodium fluorescein. Angiography of the anterior segment is of scant practical value, as it adds little to the information on the possible presence and degree of existing iris neovascularization given by slit-lamp microscopy.

Informative as they are, arterial retinal fluorescein studies constitute more of an experimental procedure; they are more difficult to perform, require hospitalization, and are safe only in experienced hands.

Fundus examination with the slit-lamp and three-mirror contact lens or a flat contact lens is always indicated. Although important as a means of achieving a passably accurate idea of the condition of the fundus as a whole, binocular indirect ophthalmoscopy cannot compare with biomicroscopy when it comes to gaining a really close view of the retina, the vitreous, or the relationship of both. A plethora of details which would otherwise escape notice is revealed. Most of the microaneurysms and distended capillaries, and even the finest epiretinal or intravitreal new vessels may easily be seen, as may any degree of retinal edema and all the existing microcystoid spaces. Similarly, detachment or thickening of the posterior hyaloid face can only be visualized with the slit-lamp, and the same may be said of the adhesions which form between the posterior hyaloid and the fibrovascular tissue that breaks through the internal limiting membrane or invades the area of Martegiani located before the disc. On the other hand, in cases of great vitreous turbidity, examination of the extreme fundus periphery with the binocular indirect ophthalmoscope and scleral indentation may show the ora and a retro-oral strip of retina, and permit the exclusion of a diagnosis of retinal detachment, at least of the rhegmatogenous type.

Gonioscopy may be of help when one is in doubt as to whether a rise in tension is due to chronic simple glaucoma or to an incipient neovascular glaucoma.

Accurate recording of all the changes detected in the fundus is obligatory if these changes and their permutations are to be assessed adequately. Fundus diagrams, with brief marginal comments, are an indispensable first step, particularly in the case of the proliferative form of the disease. Drawing in many colors on the Amsler chart is time consuming, however, and must be left in the hands of an assistant who may not always have the required skills. The cartographic documentation of the biomicroscopic changes seen through a flat contact lens could not be easier to plot whereas that of changes detected through the three-mirror lens is rather involved and requires the use of special techniques (Dufour, 1967; Plange, 1971); these allow for the one-sided specular transposition undergone by the images as they appear in the mirrors. Written descriptions of no more than 200 words by a trained observer are of great value, and should complement as a summation every patient's chart.

Color fundus photography, preferably stereoscopic photography, of some of the seven predetermined fields in the modified Airlie House classification of diabetic retinopathy is imperative if a measure of objectivity is to be achieved (Davis, 1972). Only occasionally will more than three fields have to be photographed. Even in written descriptions reference should be made to those fields. Each of the seven standard fields is approximately 30° in diameter, and corresponds to the area seen in one field when the indirect ophthalmoscope is used in conjunction with a + 14 diopter lens. Definition of the standard fields is as follows (Fig. 4-1).

Field 5: Lower edge of field tangent to a horizontal line passing through upper edge of disc, and nasal end of field tangent to a vertical line passing through center of disc.

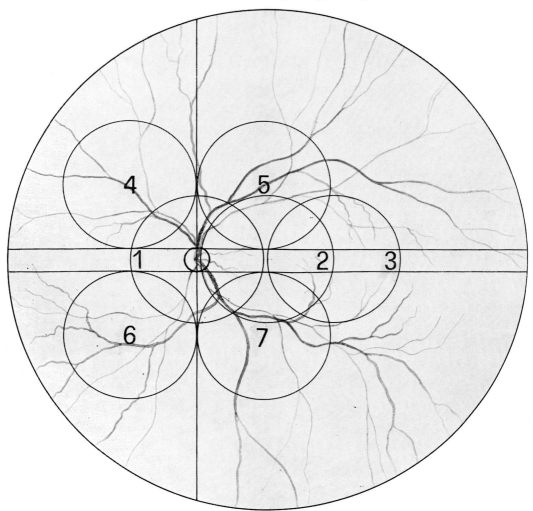

FIG. 4-1. — Standard photographic fields of the fundus as defined in the Airlie House classification (modified by Davis, 1972). For explanation see text.

Field 1: Center of optic disc at intersection of cross hairs in ocular.

Field 2: Fovea at intersection of cross hairs in ocular.

Field 3: Nasal end of horizontal cross hair at fovea.

Field 4: Lower edge of field tangent to a horizontal line passing through upper edge of the disc, and temporal edge of field tangent to a vertical line passing through center of disc.

Field 6 : Upper edge of field tangent to a horizontal line passing through lower edge of disc, and temporal edge of field tangent to a vertical line passing through center of disc.

Field 7: Upper edge of field tangent to a horizontal line passing through lower edge of disc, and nasal edge of field tangent to a vertical line passing through center of disc.

If new vessels, fibrous proliferations, or retinal breaks are present in parts of the fundus not in-

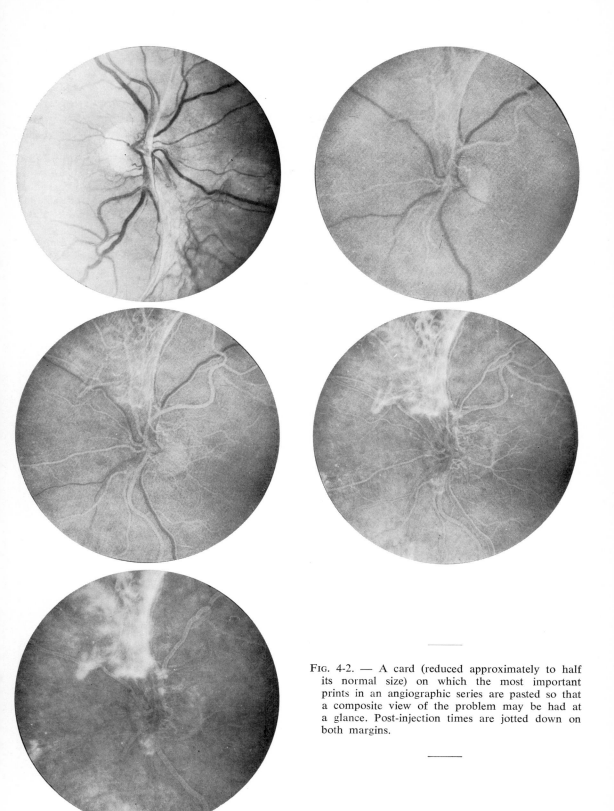

Fig. 4-2. — A card (reduced approximately to half its normal size) on which the most important prints in an angiographic series are pasted so that a composite view of the problem may be had at a glance. Post-injection times are jotted down on both margins.

cluded in the seven standard fields, additional fields should be chosen to include them. The approximate elevation of any given feature as seen by direct ophtalmoscopy should be measured in diopters or in millimeters (there are approximately 3 diopters to the millimeter), not in disc diameters as is currently being done.

In every case there is a partial overlap between fields. This can be turned to advantage when trying to specify the exact site of a lesion to be photocoagulated or excised. Thus, if somebody says that a cluster of microaneurysms lies in area 2-3, a tuft of new vessels in area 1-5, or a preretinal band in area 1-7, there remains little doubt as to where the lesion actually is. As a rule, three photographs are taken of each individual field so that two will be good even if one fails. Of these one or two will be stored and the other incorporated into the patient's personal file, together with some of the

black and white photographs taken after the intravenous injection of sodium fluorescein. In general, these will all be centered on the disc or the fovea, or on an intermediate point between them (area 1-2). For clinical use it is recommended that the mounted transparencies from each patient be preserved in clear, multi-pocketed vinyl sleeves of sufficient rigidity. When held against a viewing screen these allow excellent appraisal at a glance of the changes occuring in existing abnormalities. A few selected fluorescein prints should be pasted on a sheet of light cardboard as shown in Fig. 4-2.

Filing the photographic material poses a problem which becomes more and more complicated as the number of patients increases. A master card must be kept for each particular roll. In it will be entered the dates, the patients' names and diagnoses, the pertinent technical data, and the fields which happened to be photographed. The master cards

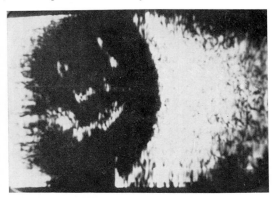

FIG. 4-3. — B-scan ultrasonogram showing a moderate amount of coagulated blood in vitreous cavity.

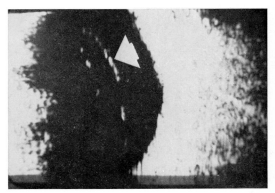

FIG. 4-4. — B-scan ultrasonogram showing a thin, veil-like sheet of fibrin in vitreous cavity. Most of the membrane lies on the posterior surface of the detached vitreous (arrow).

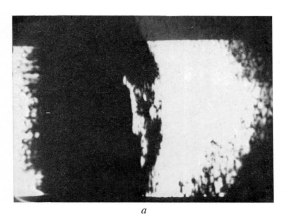

a

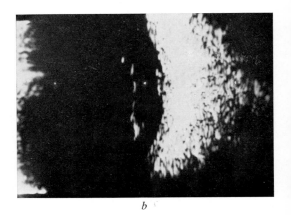

b

FIG. 4-5. — *a)* B-scan ultrasonogram showing a dense preretinal vitreous membrane. Note the linear configuration and rather distinct borders (80 dB). *b)* Same section at low gain (60 dB).

are numbered in succession and collected in three-ring binders.

An individual 7.5 × 12 cm card will then be made for each patient. In it will be listed, under the name and diagnosis, all the film rolls and numbered frames in which that patient appears. Entries in red ink refer to color photographs; entries in black to black and white photographs, including fluorescein photographs. The individual cards are placed in alphabetical order in a filing cabinet.

The slides that are held in reserve had better be kept in the cardboard or plastic containers in which they are returned by the processing laboratory. Such containers must carry the same number as the master cards to which they

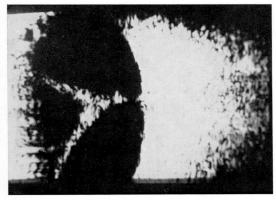

FIG. 4-6. — Dense, funnel-like membrane arising from optic nervehead. The lack of insertion directly on nerve and the thickness of the echo are not consistent with a diagnosis of retinal detachment.

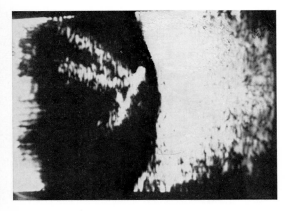

FIG. 4-7. — B-scan ultrasonogram of an eye with a thick stalk of fibrovascular tissue. The stalk diverges as it progresses forward in the vitreous compartment; it continues as a dense membrane which reaches the vitreous base.

correspond. Being in apposition with each other, the slides in the boxes are less liable to be damaged by humidity of fungal growth than they would if otherwise stored.

Other, more sophisticated methods of examination, such as ultrasonography, are indicated whenever there is a dense opacity of the optical media, the lens and vitreous in particular, if any major operation is contemplated. Both the A-mode (time-amplitude) and the B-mode (intensity modulated) echo systems yield excellent diagnostic results; they complement each other, and should be carried out simultaneously for maximal information. For all practical purposes, however, the B-mode pictures are illustrative enough, especially with the newer techniques that convert the black and white tracings into three to eight color displays. Nevertheless, I know from personal experience that correct interpretation of the pictures is far from easy, and training under the guidance of an expert is recommended.

Though unclotted blood in the vitreous is anechoic or at least difficult to capture ultrasonically, the density, mobility and degree of organization of coagulated blood are readily apparent (Fig. 4-3). Vitreous strands and sheets are usually moderate reflectors of the sound waves, but may return only faint echoes if they are insubstantial and tendril- or veil-like. The detached retina is a strong reflector, and total detachments are recognized without difficulty in that they can always be traced serially to the optic nerve. In cases of localized or flat detachments the diagnostic possibilities depend on the resolution of which the instrument is capable (Coleman, 1972; Bronson, 1973 and 1974). Ideally, ultrasound examination should enable the observer to distinguish between three different sorts of structures: (*a*) the so-called vitreous membranes, which are not really membranes in a histological sense but a (mostly hematogenous) conglomerate or condensation of fibrin and collagen fibers (Figs. 4-4 and 4-5); (*b*) the strands, stalks and sheets composed of fibrovascular tissue which are retinal in origin and result from the proliferative process (Figs. 4-6 and 4-7); and (*c*) the detached retina, which is submitted to increasing traction as both the vitreous and the proliferations shrink (Fig. 4-8). When a vitreous membrane is dense and linear and is attached to the retina near the optic nervehead, it may be hard to differentiate from a retinal detachment (Fig. 4-9). Again, diagnosis may be difficult when there are multiple parallel membranes and one can not tell for sure whether or not there is an associated retinal detachment (Fig. 4-10). Conversely, intersecting membranes are

rather easily recognized, even if located very pos-
terioly (Coleman and Franzen, 1974) (Fig. 4-11).
It is to be remembered that the space posterior to
the elevated retina is acoustically clear and appears
black on the screen (Jack *et al.,* 1974). An A-scan
display may be of help in that it indicates the
thickness of the membranes and forewarns the
surgeon of the difficulties he may run into during
the performance of vitrectomy (Freyler and Nichorlis, 1974).

In those cases where it is difficult from the
profile pattern and the echo amplitude to distinguish between a morning-glory type of detachment
and a massive proliferation arising from the disc,
bright-flash electroretinography may be of value:
it will show a large *a* wave if the retina is in place

and is not too badly damaged, but not if the retina
is detached (Figs. 4-12 and 4-13). Vitreous opacities can often be dense enough to abolish the
electrical responses of a potentially functioning
retina when this is tested in the standard way. But
few if any ocular opacities are sufficiently dense
to extinguish the bright-flash ERG if functional
retina exists behind the opacities. In most of the
eyes for which vitreous surgery is considered, the
a wave gives more useful information than does
the *b* wave. The *a* wave originates in the photo-
receptor cells and is abolished if these cells are
not functioning; in particular, the *a* wave is abolished when the retina is detached from the pigment
epithelium, or suffers from a diffuse atrophy. The
b wave is generated by the bipolar cells and is

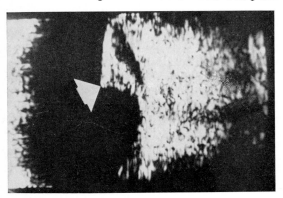

Fɪɢ. 4-8. — B-scan ultrasonogram of an eye showing a limited traction retinal detachment. A gross
proliferative mass (arrow) attaches to the retina
and protrudes into the vitreous cavity.

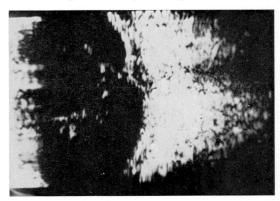

Fɪɢ. 4-10. — B-scan ultrasonogram showing both
pre- and epiretinal membranes attached to the
optic disc. The presence of an associated, flat
traction detachment could be determined at surgery.

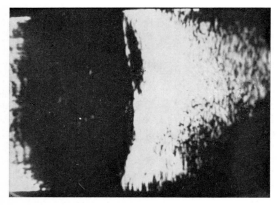

Fɪɢ. 4-9. — B-scan ultrasonogram showing a dense,
linear membrane which developed between the
upper edge of the optic nervehead and an old
photocoagulation scar. Only at surgery could this
be differentiated from a localized traction detachment.

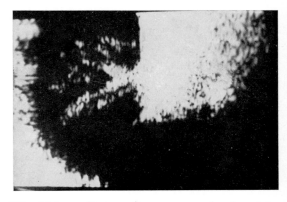

Fɪɢ. 4-11. — B-scan ultrasonogram showing dense
shadows extending forward from the optic nervehead in a typical pattern of intersecting membranes.

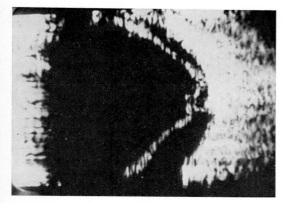

FIG. 4-12. — B-scan ultrasonogram of an eye with opaque vitreous, showing an extensive and dense single line of echoes which is connected to the optic nervehead and could correspond to a vitreous membrane or retina. Vision in this eye was light perception with poor projection.

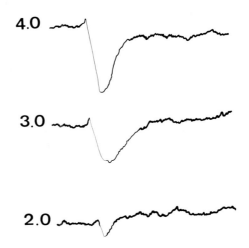

FIG. 4-13. — Bright-flash ERG of the eye shown in Fig. 4-12. Large *a* wave reveals that retina is in place; absence of *b* wave is due to the retinal changes associated with the underlying disease.

often depressed or even absent in advanced diabetic retinopathy (Fuller and Knighton, 1975).

Recording the rapid oscillatory potential in the ERG has been said to be of prognostic value in juvenile-onset diabetics, allowing anticipation of the development of proliferative changes (Simionsen, 1974).

CHAPTER 5

METABOLIC CONTROL AND DIABETIC RETINOPATHY

The regular use of the ophthalmoscope and of the retinal camera can be for the good of the patient but only if we take appropriate action; it is futile as far as he is concerned if we regard it as recording the hand of fate. This does not mean that diabetic retinopathy is always amenable to treatment; it just means that in many of its clinical forms it may be reached through one of the several avenues open to us. Therapy will obviously not reverse blindness, but it can prevent or considerably delay it when resorted to early enough. Granting that diabetes mellitus with its manifold complications and associate disorders is an incurable disease, and that to avail oneself only of symptomatic treatment is under most circumstances a far from admirable principle, there is everything to be said for taking positive steps to ensure postponement of visual loss. After all, in the face of a foreshortened life expectancy, buying time with even stopgap measures is surely worthwhile.

It should be recalled too that most medical treatment, apart from the use of antibiotics or sulfa drugs in infectious diseases, is nothing but removal of symptoms. Treatment with other drugs is aimed at replacing some element which is being produced in insufficient amounts or is altogether missing, at facilitating adjustement to an abnormal situation, or just at eliminating a single but particularly bothersome symptom, as when one gives aspirin for headache; but never — or almost never — at uprooting the cause or relieving the primary disorder.

Several controlled investigations on the relationship of retinopathy to the management of the metabolic disturbance have shown that good control of diabetes reduces the frequency or retards the appearance of retinopathy in patients with normal fundi, but does not affect the lesions once they have become manifest (Hardin *et al.*, 1956; Schlessinger *et al.*, 1960; Root, 1965, Caird, 1968; Knowles, 1968*a*; Kohner *et al.*, 1968; Burditt *et*

al., 1968; Caird *et al.*, 1968). The results of those investigations may be summarized as follows:

1. There is a positive correlation between the degree of glycosuria and the presence of retinopathy, at least in those under 60 years of age. The evidence is particularly significant in those studies where the control of diabetes is assured by means of the so-called « glycosuria percentage » (Caird, 1967).

2. Patients whose diabetes has been well controlled during the first five years after diagnosis and poorly controlled afterward do better from the ocular standpoint than those with the opposite sequence. This suggests that heavy glycosuria is more critical during the first five years of known diabetes than later in the course of the disease (Constam, 1965; Knowles, 1968*b*).

3. The absence of any clear influence of metabolic control on the evolution of even incipient retinopathy indicates that these processes are largely autonomous and independent of whatever initiated them after the earliest detectable stages. Thus, although an increase in protein-bound carbohydrate exists in the thickened basal membrane of the small blood vessels in diabetic angiopathy, it would not seem that this comes from the deposition of circulating substances.

The main point to remember appears to be that strict diabetic control plays an important role in the prevention of the angiopathy as it affects the retinal structures. In confirmation of this it should be mentioned that in the lean years during and following World War II Mehnert (1969) saw a much reduced incidence of diabetic retinopathy in continental Europe. Schöffling and Graeve (1956) noticed a considerable reduction in the severity of the macro- and microangiopathy found in autopsy material collected in Germany from 1942 to 1948 when compared to the material studied from 1948 to 1954. « The experience at the Joslin Clinic » say Bradley and Ramos (1971) « has led... to the opinion that diagnosing diabetes early and treating the patient intensively, significantly delays the development of degrees of angiopathy that are clinically threatening. In advising the physician as to the best course to follow... one can only exhort him to apply a simple principle, in the earlier (10 to 20) years of diabetes. Since the blood glucose level is the most accurate parameter of the effectiveness of insulin, in principle the one objective in treatment should be to keep this level within as normal limits as possible. This can and should (also) be insisted upon for both patients on diet and those responsive to oral hypoglycemic agents ». It has been pointed out, moreover, that it is usually diabetic persons in whom treatment has been delayed or inadequate, and in whom the diet has been improper with resulting marked hyperglycemia and glycosuria, who most frequently develop proliferative retinopathy. In the experience of Root *et al.* (1959) no patient with excellent or good diabetic control — immediate use of insulin at the onset of diabetes, continuous medical supervision, and daily testing of the urine — has been seen to suffer from proliferative retinopathy. This point, however, may not be widely agreed upon. In fact, it seems to me that the duration and control of diabetes are much more closely related to the occurrence and severity of background retinopathy than to the occurrence and severity of proliferative retinopathy.

Once the retinopathy has set in there is little one can expect from even the strictest regulation of dietary factors and systemic medical surveillance. The numerical study of Caird and Garret (1963) already referred to failed to show any difference in the rate of progression of both visual deterioration and established retinopathy between patients with good and patients with poor control of their diabetes; it showed instead that no reliance can be placed on control of diabetes to prevent visual impairment due to retinopathy. The claim by Kohner *et al.* (1968) that very good diabetic control seems to protect patients with an overt retinopathy from a multiplication of the existing microaneurysms, hemorrhages and new vessels, although not from a worsening of exudates or of the glial, proliferative changes, may find an explanation in the fact that their patient with very good control were mostly adult-onset diabetics with a more favorable prognosis *.

The above view takes for granted that the diffuse thickening of the capillary basement membrane follows and does not precede the carbohydrate intolerance, and that diabetic microangiopathy is a consequence of hyperglycemia rather than the result of a predisposition to angiopathy which is separately determined and is not part of the diabetic state. It cannot even be reconciled with the view that the microangiopathy is an integral component of the disease itself. Such a hypothesis, which is naturally the simplest, has not always been substantiated by facts. Thus, to cite but one observation which casts some doubts as to the exclusive role of hyperglycemia in the production of diabetic retinopathy, one may recall that after pituitary ablation followed by an improved fundus picture, therapy is directed toward maintaining a persistent hyperglycemia in an effort to parry the ever present risk of hypoglycemia to which these patient are prone.

And yet the fact that good control seems to inhibit to some degree the development of vascular changes, that an angiopathy appears in secondary diabetes, and also that lesions very similar to diabetic angiopathy can be produced regularly in the kidney of alloxanized rats and dogs with severe diabetes goes to show unequivocally (*a*) that heredity is not necssary for the development of microangiopathy, (*b*) that the severity of the metabolic disturbance is important in this respect, and (*c*) that meticulous attention to control can prevent or significantly reduce the angiopathy of diabetes (Lundbaek *et al.*, 1970; Bloodworth and Engerman, 1973).

But since prevention of the retinopathy through the control of diabetes is only relative in that good control merely reduces the frequency and severity or retards the advent of the fundus changes, one must conclude that there is more to the pathogenesis of the microangiopathy than solely the disturbance of the carbohydrate metabolism. If the patients live long enough, a large number of them will come to suffer from at least some sort of ocular complication, however strict the dietary and therapeutic regimen to which they have been submitted and however ready they are to cooperate. Hence the unremitting search for newer and more reliable methods to combat the established retinal malady.

_____

* If hypersecretion of growth hormone is indeed a critical causal factor in the development of diabetic angiopathy as suggested by Lundbaek *et al* (1971) and if, in some patients at least, improved control lowers the plasma growth hormone concentration even in children as shown by Baird *et al.* (1973), one would expect that the routine management of the metabolic disturbance is not without influence on the course of established retinopathy. The reason for the discrepancy between this postulate and the results of clinical observation is not clear.

CHAPTER 6

MEDICAL TREATMENT OF DIABETIC RETINOPATHY

The best critical survey of the numerous medications that have been used at one time or another for diabetic retinopathy is that of Bradley and Ramos (1971). As a fresh inquiry into the subject would only be repetitive and pointless, the reader is referred to their original description for details. Thus we shall confine the present discussion to those measures that have proved of indisputable efficacy, to a review of the few properly randomized trials controlled for patient and observer variation, and to the latest contributions which, by being based on sound premises, seem to afford ground for reasonable expectations.

In the nonproliferative type of retinopathy, the treatments proposed so far have been directed at preventing the onset of the proliferative stage or at achieving a resolution of the macular involvement by edema and fatty circinate complexes.

In the particular case of *exudative maculopathy,* there is ample evidence to substantiate the claim that lowering the circulating lipids has a favorable effect on the retinal lesions, if not necessarily on central vision. It is certain that the hard or waxy exudates contain fat, the fatty material being partly intra- and partly extracellular; and it seems definitely established that a reduction of serum cholesterol, triglycerides or the general blood lipid concentration — either through qualitative dietary control aimed at reducing the intake of fat, or through the employment of different drugs — is conducive to an amelioration of the retinal lesions.

Kempner *et al.* (1958), VanEck (1959), and Ernest *et al.* (1965) have noted a marked decrease in the extent and even a disappearance of hard exudates in patients submitted to a diet low in animal fat, though not a corresponding amelioration of the vascular lesions. More important is the assay designed by King *et al.* (1963) to determine the effect of a corn-oil diet on the mobility of the macular exudates: 23 patients (37 eyes) continued with their normal saturated fat consumption while 17 (26 eyes) limited their daily ingestion to 20 g with the adidtion of 60 g of unsaturated vegetable fat. The serum lipid levels fell in most of the treated patients, with some variations. In the treated group there was a marked reduction in the amount and size of the retinal exudates. Favorable changes in the extent of hemorrhage were also observed, but only in those patients who had a significant drop in blood pressure during the observation period. If it is disappointing to record that no significant associated recovery in visual acuity took place, one must keep in mind that the exudates are regarded as both the consequence and the cause of neuronal destruction. In any event, it may be well to realize that the institution of these or similar diets may well arrest further functional deterioration.

Among the many pharmacological agents that have been tried with the same end in view, heparin given sublingually or parenterally because of its supposedly clearing effect on the larger, less dense fat molecules has been credited with an ability to lower the extent and number of the retinal deposits (Finley and Weaver, 1960; Finley, 1961). Based on my own findings, however, and on the fact that the above were not adequately controlled trials, I believe that there is little evidence to support the claim that heparin can be of use in the prevention or treatment of the exudative phenomena. The same may be said of the salicylates, mainly in the form of para-aminosalicylic acid in large doses, in spite of their possible influence on the serum cholesterol, total lipid, and phospholipid levels (Esman *et al.,* 1963; Mooney, 1963). On the other hand the value of clofibrate, or ethyl-chlorophenoxyisobutyrate, either alone (Atromid-S) or in combination with androsterone (Atromid) in reducing the plasma concentration of cholesterol, triglycerides, and other lipoid fractions, and in improving retinal exudates has been demonstrated beyond the shadow of a doubt. At least five well-designed therapeutic trials bear out this statement (Cullen *et al.*, 1964; Duncan *et al.*, 1968; Houtsmuller, 1968; Harold *et al.*, 1969; Regnault *et al.*, 1970; Cullen *et al.*, 1974).

It would appear, therefore, that in the case of exudative maculopathy in the maturity-onset diabetic, an effort should be made to keep the patient on a diet poor in animal fat (10-20 g per day) and moderately rich in unsaturated vegetal fat (60 g per day). The addition of the unsaturated fat is necessary if one wishes to avoid the increase in carbohydrate intake which would otherwise be required to prevent weight loss. Clofibrate at a daily dosage of 2 g for prolonged periods of time should also be recommended. But although some resorption of fatty exudates can be brought about in this way, both the above diet and the clofibrate have no effect on increased permeability with the resulting retinal edema and cystoid degeneration of the macula.

Treatment of the *congestive and hemorrhagic* form of nonproliferative retinopathy with carbazochrome and with anticoagulants such as coumarin derivatives — to reduce capillary permeability, increase capillary resistance, and avoid arteriolar occlusion, venous distension and circulatory sludginess in the retinal vasculature — has been shown to be nugatory by the studies of Keeney and Mody (1955) and of Valdorf-Hansen *et al.* (1969). The reason for the use of the nonandrogenic anabolic steroids, of estrogens or testosterone, and of vitamin B_{12}, is not clear. In any event the double blind controlled trial by Hunter *et al.* (1967) with anabolic steroids yielded entirely negative results as did the carefully constructed study with vitamin B_{12} by Keen and Smith (1959).

Among the drugs that have been recommended of late, few appear to be promising. One such is calcium dobesilate (Doxium) which possesses a well-documented antihemorrhagic activity. Sévin and Cuendet (1969*a* and *b*), Bisantis (1971) and Németh *et al.* (1975) have clearly shown that this substance is capable of restoring capillary resistance — which is markedly diminished in the diabetic patient with retinopathy when measured by means of a suction cup applied to the bulbar conjunctiva — to its normal value of 35 cm Hg; they have also shown that upon the cessation of treatment the capillary resistance returns to its initial abnormally low level.

In this respect, it should be pointed out that the ultrastructure of the conjunctival capillaries closely matches that of the retinal capillaries (Regnault *et al.*, 1970) and that the vascular changes in the conjunctiva compare with those in the retina to a certain degree (Eisalo and Raitta, 1971).

Clinically, the results obtained by the same authors in a large series of patients have been encouraging in that the detectable retinal hemorrhages of simple retinopathy diminished rapidly in number after six months of treatment with Doxium, and tended to disappear after 18 months. By using a special method with fluorescence angiography to quantitate the amount of leakage from microaneurysms and abnormal intraretinal capillaries, Sévin and Cuendet (1971) were able to prove that the same drug exerts a favorable influence upon augmented capillary permeability. Although no control series was set up, statistical analysis of the results obtained revealed that the hemorrhages underwent a considerable reduction after treatment, and that a parallelism existed between the enhanced capillary resistance and the correction of the abnormal diffusion through the vascular walls. In passing, it should be noted that the antiexudative effect of this compound is less evident than its antihemorrhagic effect, and that its influence upon the large hard exudates is far from impressive (Offret et Guyot, 1972).

An oral dose of 250 mg of Doxium given twice to four times daily for 4 consecutives months seems to be average for restoring the capillary resistance and permeability to normal. A daily maintenance dose of 250 mg is then needed to consolidate the results. No undesirable side effects have been reported.

It has been assumed that this synthetic derivative owes its dual antihemorrhagic and antiexudative properties to its action upon the adhesive and aggregative capacity of the platelets (Sévin, 1971).

In spite of the initially encouraging results, a word of caution should be advanced in view of the limited duration of the experience collected so far, and of the scarcity of truly randomized studies with reasonable design and control. Quite recently, however, Freyler and Sehorst (1974) have conducted a double blind trial on 48 patients with simple diabetic retinopathy which shows that calcium dobesilate possesses a statistically significant effect on the increased permeability of the retinal capillaries. Leakage, as demonstrated by fluorescein angiography, was chosen as a main criterion in assessing the angiotropic properties of the drug. In a further investigation Freyler (1974) showed that normalization of permeability brought about a regression of the retinal lesions.

The use of pyrimidyl-piperonyl-piperazine (Trivastal) for the purpose of augmenting the blood supply to peripheral areas would seem to be rational, if one remembers that recent work by Garner and Ashton (1972) has shown that the mean area of the ophthalmic artery ostium in subjects with diabetic retinopathy is only 0.58 mm^2, whereas in those cases without retinopathy it is 0.96 mm^2, the difference being statistically significant ($p < 0.005$). This supports the view that reduced blood flow to the retina may be a factor in the pathogenesis of retinopathy and that, if it is questionable whether ischemia is of importance in initiating the fundus changes, it is now quite certain that it plays a role in their natural course (cf. p. 9). Unfortunately, the results reported by Arion *et al.* (1969) with this drug failed to prove that it has any beneficial effects.

Pyridinolcarbamate (Duaxol) has been tried by some with the aim of preventing the impaired perfusion resulting from arteriolar involvement in diabetic retinopathy. In a non-controlled study, Takaku *et al.* (1969) reported good results in 40 cases of variable severity. Offret *et al.* (1969) think differently, as does this writer, who has conducted a controlled trial in 60 cases, of which 30 were treated and 30 were left untreated, and who found no difference between the two groups after an 18-month interval.

Once the condition has reached the *proliferative stage,* no known form of conservative therapy is of any avail. As could be expected from the fact that the new vessels have practically no basal membrane and are therefore highly permeable and weak, the response to the administration of calcium dobesilate is poor in that it does not succeed in halting the recurring intravitreal hemorrhages. Antimetabolites such as azathioprine (Imuran) have been used by Houtsmuller (1972) in a small number of cases with irregular results.

The latter author feels that the successful attempts made recently by Kolodny *et al.* (1971) in acromegaly to inhibit growth hormone formation with chlorpromazine (Thorazine, Ampliactil) — a nonsteroidal phenothiazine derivative which depresses the hypothalamus — and with medroxyprogesterone offer some hope of pharmacologically controlling diabetic retinopathy. In my experience, unfortunately, this has not been the case, for chlorpromazine remained without effect on the fundus picture of 12 juvenile diabetics with proliferative retinopathy of variable severity after being given orally for 60 days at the recommended dosage of 25 mg four times a day. In this connection it should be pointed out that Singh *et al.* (1973) found that plasma growth hormone was unaffected by chlorpromazine in six acromegalic patients. Medroxyprogesterone acetate also

failed to influence the fundus picture in another ten similarly affected cases, even though it did markedly lower HGH concentration (and brought about reversible impotence in the male and amenorrhea in the female) during a 40-day course of therapy when the drug was administered by mouth in a daily dose of 40 mg. A fall of basal plasma levels of growth hormone was observed by Liuzzi *et al.* (1972) after medroxyprogesterone administration in acromegalic patients; none of them, however, had the levels fall to normal.

It may well be that in the future *somatostatin,* a peptide inhibiting somatotrophin release that has been isolated from crude hypothalamic extracts by Brazeau *et al.* (1973) will prove to be of clinical significance in the treatment of juvenile diabetics, with of without retinopathy. The onset of the inhibiting action of somatostatin is extremely rapid and its biological half-life extremely short in animals and in man. A long-acting preparation of somatostatin would thus be necessary for clinical use (Brazeau *et al.,* 1974). Meissner *et al.* (1975) are of the opinion that the suppression of the secretion of growth hormone and glucacon, both insulin antagonists, is responsible for the antidiabetic action of somatostatin.

As it is, all that can be done is to help the patient with a regimen and advice aimed at reducing the risk, the frequency, and the importance of hemorrhaging. A regimen for permanent control, whether diet, oral hypoglycemic agents, or insulin, should avoid hypoglycemia in patients with retinal neovascularization, especially those who have already suffered from bleeding episodes. Because of its ability to provoke a higher secretion rate of growth hormone, sudden or sustained hypoglycemia is inquestionably a major factor in instigating hemorrhage in such patients. Likewise systolic and particularly diastolic hypertension should be kept under the 100 mm Hg mark as they are both associated with a tendency toward recurring hemorrhage. Hence, frequent checkups by the internist are necessary.

In so far as hygienic measures conducive to the prevention of bleeding go, the patient should most carefully avoid any thoracic or cephalic congestion which would create an abrupt change in pressure within the retinal vessels. Without being confined to a sedentary life, he should be required to avoid excessive cardiac work, as denoted by the onset of dyspnea during the performance of physical activity. Since expenditure of energy involved in carrying out individual chores cannot be measured accurately, the patient's own subjective responses to effort must be the guide in determining the nature and extent of his limitations. Immoderate exercise should also be avoided for the simple reason that it tends to produce an abnormal rise in the plasma level of growth hormone even in the well-controlled diabetic (Lundbaek *et al.,* 1970).

Some say that the head should be kept raised at all times, and that the headboard of the bed should be raised by 20 to 30°, or two pillows used at night. No data have been presented to show that this is necessary or even helpful, however. Strain of any kind, such as may result from lifting a heavy object, must be interdicted; so must bending, jumping, holdging one's breath, and any other movement or practice likely to result in augmented intrathoracic pressure against a closed glottis. Stool softeners such as mineral oil ought to be ordered if necessary, as well as cough syrups or antihistamines if bronchial catarrh, allergic symptoms or even a common cold are present; it should be pointed out, however, that the use of nasal drops, sprays, inhalators or other medications capable of raising the blood pressure is to be shunned unless specifically indicated. The patient must be told never to blow his nose forcefully, as this would inevitably have a Valsalva effect. He should also refrain from ascending to altitudes of over 2000 m. Agitation and anxiety should be fought with tranquilizers and sedatives in doses suited to the particular case, or psychiatric counseling sought. Indeed, it can be affirmed that the effect of emotional stress or any jolting experience upon the metabolic control and the retinal vascular disease may be nefarious, this being due in all probability to a diencephalic disturbance, since the hypothalamus controls and regulates the secretion of somatotrophin through the release of a hypophysiotropic factor.

For more than one reason, pregnancy should be terminated in the eighth month by cesarean section (cf. chapter 10).

On the grounds that there is less retinopathy in diabetics with primary-open-angle glaucoma (Grafe, 1924; Christiansson, 1965; Marré and Marré, 1968), that hypotony tends to aggravate the proliferative phase of the disease (Igersheimer, 1944) and that ocular hypertension may retard the development of proliferative retinopathy, or reduce the risk of bleeding from existing new vessels, it has been suggested that steroid-induced glaucoma may be beneficial as it reduces the differential between the intracapillary pressure and the intravitreal pressure across the capillary wall (Gills and Anderson, 1969). But since adult diabetic patients with proliferative retinopathy resemble nondiabetics in their intraocular pressure reaction to topical corticosteroids, with only 10% being high responders, the number of those who may profit from the regular instillation of these drugs is limited (Becker *et al.,* 1966; Becker, 1971). As noted by Graham (1972) there is also some conflicting evidence as to the alleged connection between diabetes mellitus and glaucoma. While it was reported by Gavey (1966) that diabetes was conspicuous by its rarity among 300 glaucomatous patients, and more recently by Bouzas *et al.* (1971) that the mean intraocular pressure of diabetics does not differ significantly from that of the normal population, Chervin *et al.* (1973) have found abnormally elevated pressures in 26.9 % of all diabetics.

Should a vitreous hemorrhage occur, pinhole spectacles or binocular occlusion with bed rest in a semierect position ought to be ordered for a week or two, until the bleeding stops and both fibrin and the cellular elements settle inferiorly. In the cases when the blood collects in the fluid-filled space between the detached posterior hyaloid and the internal limiting membrane, this will cause clearing in a remarkably short time; but in those where blood infiltrates solid vitreous in front of the hyaloid surface, settling or resorption can take months or may never occur.

CHAPTER 7

PITUITARY ABLATION

Seldom in the history of medicine has a procedure as daring and full of far-reaching consequences as hypophysectomy for diabetic retinopathy evolved out of so few and such uncertain theoretical premises. More than 40 years ago, Houssay and Biassotti (1930, 1931) showed that removal of the pituitary gland brought about an amelioration in the diabetic state of pancreatectomized dogs in which no retinopathy existed. Shortly afterward Lyall and Innes (1935) described the Houssay phenomena in man. The striking observation of Poulsen concerning a 30-year-old woman whose malignant retinopathy regressed following abortion complicated by pituitary necrosis (Sheehan's syndrome) did not come until 1953. Even before that time, on such flimsy evidence as was available to them, Luft et al. (1952, 1955a and b) had begun trying to influence diabetic angiopathy, and more specifically recurring retinal and vitreous hemorrhages, by hypophysectomy. Until quite recently, however, no definite proof existed that pituitary ablation favorably affects the course of the retinopathy, so that the procedure remained without foundation for years.

Young (1937) and Houssay and Rodríguez (1953) demonstrated the direct diabetogenic action of various preparations of growth hormone in the laboratory; Ikkos and Luft (1960) observed that growth hormone showed a similar effect when injected in man. Only after the introduction of radioimmunological techniques for measuring the level of growth hormone in plasma could an answer be given to the question of whether the serum hormone level was high in the diabetic patient during ordinary life. To the best of my knowledge, Hansen and Johansen (1969) were the first to demonstrate that in patients with classic juvenile diabetes the values obtained through a 24-hour period are much higher than in the nondiabetic, and that in the former the curve is characterized by frequent and steep peaks. According to the same authors, the mean serum growth hormone level of nondiabetics was 1.98 ng/ml, and that of juvenile diabetics 7.26 ng/ml, that is, three to four times higher. Lundbaek et al. (1970) obtained similar results.

Using Yalow and Berson's (1968) method of assay, Sévin (1972a) made the important observation that, in diabetic subjects with proliferative retinopathy whose lesions remained stable or presented only slow deterioration, the plasma concentration of growth hormone ranged from 0.5 to 5.4 ng/ml in men, and from 0.65 to 6.2 ng/ml in women; in patients with marked deterioration, the figures went from 0.90 up to 35 ng/ml; and in those who improved they fell from 23.6 to 0.60 in a few weeks' time. Working independently, Frezzoti et al. (1972) obtained comparable results, as did Knopf et al. (1972) who found fasting HGH levels to be higher in diabetic than in normal persons, and higher still in diabetic persons with retinopathy than in those without retinopathy. This lends strong support to the view that growth hormone is, if not the cause, at least a major factor in the development of proliferative diabetic retinopathy (see p. 53). It may be said that an abnormal concentration of growth hormone can, and does, worsen the picture of established proliferative retinopathy even if it is not responsible for the appearance of retinal neovascularization, just as in the case of the nonproliferative form, impairment from repeated and copious hemorrhagic episodes is often dependent upon the presence of atheromatous changes, high blood pressure, or both (Sévin, 1972b), even though these are not basically the cause.

Further support for the concept of the importance of growth hormone comes from Merimee et al. (1970) who drew attention to the fact that no microangiopathy develops in diabetic dwarfs with a much diminished monotrophic hypophyseal function. Evidence to the contrary is feeble and consists solely of the comparative rarity of retinopathy in diabetes secondary to acromegaly, where there is oversecretion of that hormone over a long period of time (McCullagh, 1956; Powell et al., 1966).

Even though a large number of earlier papers had suggested that pituitary ablation was indeed capable of arresting and even partially reversing advanced diabetic retinopathy, one had to wait for the report of Ray et al. (1968) to get a long-term evaluation of the results obtained in a large series of cases. A randomized trial was conducted by Lundbaek et al. (1968) in two well-matched groups of patients suffering from retinopathy — not always proliferative — of variable severity, of whom 15 were totally hypophysectomized through the transsphenoidal route and 15 kept as controls. After an observation period of one to five years it could be seen that progression of the prolifera-tive changes was more common in the controls than in the operated patients, as was progression of rubeosis iridis when present. No conspicuous difference could be observed, however, on other lesions such as microaneurysms, hemorrhages, phlebopathy, edema and exudates. Periods of regression were often followed by periods of reactivation in both the hypophysectomized patients and the controls.

Therefore, it appears from this study that if pituitary ablation affords some protection against the malignant ocular manifestations of diabetic angiopathy, it is ineffective against background retinopathy.

The other prospective trial where two sets of patients with similar initial gradings were compared is that by Kohner et al. (1972). In 26, pituitary destruction was performed by yttrium-90 implan-tation; 26 were used as controls. New vessel for-mation was not necessary for consideration of pituitary irradiation. Both groups of patients were followed for five years or more. Treated patients fared significantly better at all times than the controls, the difference being due to improvement in those who were treated rather than to deterio-ration in the control group. The data presented indicate that pituitary suppression exerted a salu-tary effect which consisted not only in an arrest of new vessel formation but in actual regression. Microaneurysms, hemorrhages, venous abnormal-ities, and the visual acuity were also seen to react favorably. Macular edema and hard exudates remained unaltered, however, as did fibrous pro-liferation. Nevertheless, as will be shown presently, one cannot accept without reservation the conclud-ing remark by these authors that new vessels on the disc, in patients who are otherwise suitable, remain an almost absolute indication for complete pituitary ablation if blindness is to be avoided. Although, to be sure, their study proves that the operated subjetcs did better than the controls, this may have been so because the latter were only exceptionally treated with xenon photocoagulation, and never with argon laser photocoagulation.

At present, we are left with only a very few potential candidates for hypophysectomy. These are patients who either have new vessels arising from the disc or a florid epiretinal neovasculariza-tion in both eyes, or in the one remaining sal-vageable eye, in whom light coagulation cannot be used or has proved ineffectual, and in whom the level of serum growth hormone is consistently elevated. As a rule, only patients with recurring hemorrhagic activity or with a proliferative angio-pathy advancing at such a pace that loss of central vision seems imminent are considered for ablation. Kohner et al. (1976) have shown conclusively that in the so-called « florid proliferative retinopathy » (which has been defined by them as that form of juvenile retinopathy where there is new-vessel for-mation equal to or worse than Hammersmith Hos-pital Standard C in two or more 30° photographic fields, excluding that centered on the disc) pitui-tary ablation remains the treatment of choice.

Retinal changes which constitute contraindica-tions include massive or even moderate fibrous pro-liferation, with or without retinal detachment, even if the visual acuity is still preserved; bilateral, irreversible macular damage; massive vitreous bleeding precluding adequate examination of the posterior pole; and, on the other hand, lesions of a purely edematous and exudative nature involv-ing predominantly the central region.

The accepted criteria for the selection of patients from a general standpoint are as follows (Fraser, 1966; Deckert et al., 1967; Bradley and Rees, 1968): The patients must be in fair health and reasonably controlled as regards their metabolic disturbance; have no gross impairment of renal function (blood urea under 50 mg per ml; serum creatinine under 2 mg per 100 ml; serum albumin over 3 g per 100 ml; erythrocyte sedimentation rate under 25 mm after one hour; proteinuria under 1 g per 24 hours *); have had no extensive or recent myocardial infarction; be free from arrhythmia, angina pectoris, cardiomegaly, overt or borderline cardiac failure, persistent diastolic blood pressure of 100 mm Hg or more, incapacitat-ing peripheral or visceral neuropathy, and chronic

---

* In the presence of sustained proteinuria the survival time is so short that hypophysectomy is hardly warranted.

ineradicable infection, particularly of the urinary tract. The patients must also be psychologically stable, anxious for surgery, and capable of carefully managing replacement therapy. Subjects over 45 years of age are now generally excluded.

Among the procedures for pituitary suppression that have been advocated over the years the following continue to be employed: transfrontal and transsphenoidal resection; pituitary stalk section; external, conventional roentgentherapy; transcutaneous irradiation with heavy particles, such as the proton beam, utilizing the Bragg-Peak effect; interstitial irradiation through the insertion of yttrium-90 rods; radiofrequency (stereotactic) coagulation; transsphenoidal or transethmoidal cryocoagulation. The least hazardous operatives techniques are stalk section and the various types of transnasal hypophysectomy. Although the postoperative mortality rate following the implantation of radiactive

depression, graded as complete, intermediate, and slight from endocrine tests conducted after a three-month interval (Joplin *et al.*, 1965, 1967; Adams *et al.*, 1974). Patients are considered to be totally ablated if they are both thyroid and steroid dependent, if their insuline requirements fall by 50 % or more, or if they develop amenorrhea or become impotent. Slight ablation is recorded when there is no steroid and thyroid dependency, no alteration in sexual function, and when insulin requirements fall by less than 50 %. Intermediate ablation is that in which the pituitary insufficiency varies between these extremes. There has been little in my experience to support the claim by Field (1968) that with the available substitutive preparations, self-management of hypopituitarism is surprisingly simple.

By and large, it can be said that rapid clearing of vitreous opacity, structural improvement (in

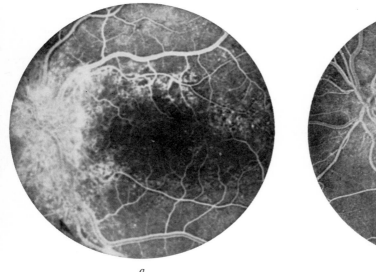 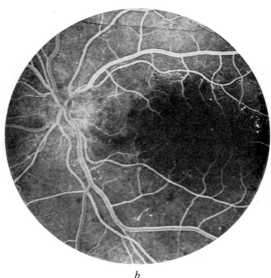

a   b

Fig. 7-1. — *a*) Fluorescein angiogram of a diabetic patient with profuse neovascularization from the disc, multiple microaneurysms, and several scattered areas of capillary closure. *b*) Considerable regression following hypophysectomy. (Courtesy Dr. L. M. Aiello.)

yttrium appears to be lower than after surgical excision, and the incidence of damage to the cerebral vessels and intracranial nerves practically negligible, cerebrospinal fluid rhinorrea and even death by meningitis have been reported in a number of cases.

It is well known that the retinal neovascular response and the reduction in the propensity to bleed are closely related to the extent of pituitary

the form of a reduction of venous caliber and segmental irregularity, lessened retinal and preretinal hemorrhagic activity, decreased leakage as revealed by serial fluorescein fundus photography, and atrophy of the new vessel systems) as well as visual amelioration may be expected to occur after complete suppression (Fig. 7-1). A similar trend, though less marked, is seen after intermediate ablation, while no change can be detected in patients with slight ablation. Patients under 40 years of age at the time of the operation benefit more than those over 40 (Oakley *et al.,* 1968; Panisset *et al.,* 1971).

From a review of the pertinent literature, it would seem that the retinopathy may be improved in about one-third of all cases, that it continues to deteriorate — although at a slower pace — in one third, and that it shows no appreciable change in the remainder. Vision can usually be preserved over five years in about 75 % of the eyes. From the few series with a follow-up of more than one or two years, it appears that the long-term results tend to parallel the initial response. It should be pointed out that Fraser *et al.* (1973) have found a disturbingly high incidence of late cardiovascular or renal deaths, and of hypertension and increased uremia among their ablated patients followed for five years or more (Fig. 7-2).

As has been pointed out by Wise *et al.* (1971), the possibility of improvement after pituitary ablation must be balanced against the risks and disadvantages of the procedure; more important, it must be weighed against the possibility of achieving

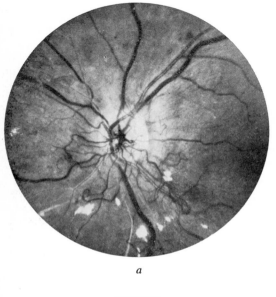

a

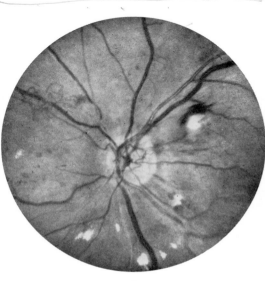

b

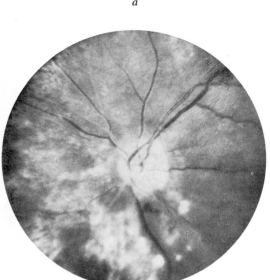

c

FIG. 7-2. — *a*) Left eye of a 38-year-old patient with diabetes of 17 years duration. There is surface disc neovascularization spreading over the surrounding retina. *b*) On year after adequate (maximal) pituitary supression. The neovascularization has been lessened but not eliminated. Uremia (75 mg/100 ml) and hypertension (180/110) have developed, and a soft exudate may be seen in the upper temporal quadrant near the disc. *c*) Total regression of the neovascularization, deturgescence of the retinal veins and disappearance of the soft exudate was achieved through extensive argon laser photocoagulation (photograph taken two years after the completion of treatment).

at least comparable results with photocoagulation, which entails virtually no risks and does not demand from the patient a willingness to become an invalid for life. Considering that the reprieve from the threat to vision is uncertain, and that impairment of renal function along with progression of coronary and peripheral vascular disease have been observed following the procedure, it would seem that to reach a decision in favor of hypophyseal destruction is no small matter, especially in the young. In fact it may demand from the patient no less resignation than does the acceptance of blindness. And yet despite its limitations there can be no doubt that pituitary supression constitutes a legitimate and effective procedure when performed in young subjects without nephropathy and without serious circulatory disturbances. It may be that its chief advantage lies in the fact that its effects on the neovascular component of the retinopathy are more durable than those of photocoagulation, which brings only a temporary respite in many cases.

It has been assumed that the removal of some hormonal pituitary factor or combination of factors explains the amelioration in the retinopathy in patients with lowered hypophyseal function. The postmortem study by Poulsen (1966) of his famous patient confirmed that a close anatomical relationship existed between the arrest of her retinopathy and necrosis of the anterior lobe of the hypophysis. It has been only lately, however, that conclusive data have been advanced in support of the theory that growth hormone is the critical agent eliminated. Wright *et al.* (1969) have shown that in 20 patients with severe pituitary suppression the maximum growth hormone level was below 2 ng/ml; in eight patients with moderate suppression there were two with similar levels, whereas in the other six these varied between 3.1 and 18 (mean, 10.5). The 11 slightly ablated patients had levels which measured between 4.2 and 32 ng/ml.

Though growth hormone is known to be an insulin antagonist, its role as a vasoformative agent seems to be unrelated to the imbalance it helps create in the carbohydrate metabolism. Were this not so, the effectiveness of pituitary ablation would be no greater than that of meticulous diabetic control. It is worth noting that Beaumont *et al.* (1971) have suggested that an excessive secretion of growth hormone could bring about diabetic capillary disease by inhibiting the metabolism of glucose, with a resulting accumulation of sorbitol within the capillary wall and consequent damage to the basement membrane. In a more general frame of reference, one should note that while somatotrophin undoubtely has a diabetogenic effect, it is not a primary factor in the development of diabetes mellitus, the present concept being that it is diabetogenic to the extent that the beta cells of the pancreas suffer from an inability to produce insulin in an adequate manner (Luft and Guillemin, 1974). Direct evidence of the relationship between an increase in plasma somatotrophin and the occurrence of diabetic vascular disease is still lacking, but indirect evidence such as has been cited above and is being supplied in chapter 8 is, I believe, categorical. As in the case of its influence on the disturbance in carbohydrate metabolism it would appear that HGH in normal or increased amounts plays a role in causing microangiopathy only in the event of defective insulin production.

Wolter and Knoblich (1965) have shown that unmyelinated fibers are present in optic nerve stumps many years after bilateral enucleation, and that some of them come from the pituitary stalk. The presence of such fibers connecting pituitary stalk and eye suggests that a neural mechanism may play a role in the improvement of diabetic retinopathy after either hypophysectomy or pituitary stalk section, particularly the latter, in which the gland itself is spared. It is well known, of course, that in stalk section the interruption of the long portal vessels leads occasionally to an infarction of the anterior lobe resulting in various degrees of hormonal insufficiency (Hardy *et al.,* 1968).

OTHER, LESS COMMON APPROACHES
TO THE PROBLEM
OF DIABETIC RETINOPATHY

Unlike photocoagulation and hypophysectomy, which are of definite value in the treatment of diabetic retinopathy despite our lack of knowledge of the pathogenesis of the condition, a number of other procedures have been used that have failed to stand the test of carefully controlled study. Among these should be mentioned adrenalectomy, radiotherapy of the posterior segment and the surgical excision of the submaxillary salivary glands.

Adrenalectomy

If adrenalectomy happens to be mentioned here at all as a treatment for advanced diabetic retinopathy, it is only to point out that it has been abandoned as futile. First the question of whether or not adrenocortical function is increased in the presence of clinically evident microangiopathy is far from settled. Secondly, adrenalectomy necessitates replacement of the hormones that one is trying to eliminate.

There are also the facts (*a*) that both Addison's disease and diabetic retinopathy have been reported in the same patient, (*b*) that diabetic retinopathy is extremely rare in individuals with Cushing's syndrome and in those who have received steroids for long periods of time, and (*c*) that the retinopathy may continue to progress after the adrenal glands have been removed (McCullagh, 1965; Beaven *et al.*, 1959; Lourie *et al.*, 1962, Oosterhuis *et al.*, 1963; Caird *et al.*, 1968; Bradley and Ramos, 1971).

Radiotherapy of the posterior segment

The same may be said of radiotherapy of the eye, since Larsen (1959) has reported on a controlled trial in two series of cases with proliferative retinopathy where the course of the disease was found to be the same in both the treated and the untreated groups after a period of 21 months.

Ablation of the salivary glands

On the grounds that the submandibular salivary glands may produce an anti-insulin-acting hormone, Godlowski *et al.* (1961) and later Motta *et al.* (1971) have suggested that ablation of these glands — and perhaps also of the sublingual glands — should act favourably upon the carbohydrate metabolism and improve the retinal changes. Some 25 cases have been operated upon so far. Although amelioration in both vision and the anatomic condition of the fundus has been reported, the results are not entirely convincing and need confirmation before this can be considered a valid mode of treatment.

CHAPTER 8

PHOTOCOAGULATION

Initially the purpose of photocoagulation was to obliterate some of the individual features of diabetic retinopathy such as microaneurysms and new vessel networks as a means of averting the risk of vitreous hemorrhage. It was subsequently thought that the favorable effect of the procedure was largely due to the destruction of normal tissue — or of hypoxic but not overtly diseased tissue — thereby reducing the metabolic activity of the retina (Meyer-Schwickerath, 1959; Wetzig and Worlton, 1963; Schott, 1964; Okun and Cibis, 1966; Wetzig and Jepson, 1966, 1968; Meyer-Schwickerath and Schott, 1968; Wessing, 1972; Riaskoff, 1972).

Thus, a highly selective approach aimed at the deletion of visible lesions gave way to a procedure less critical from a topographic standpoint, where a vast number of burns scattered over the extramacular retina tend to create a condition similar to that found in high myopia, disseminated chorioiditis, diffuse chorioretinal degeneration and extensive diathermy fundus scarring, which all seem to prevent the development of diabetic retinopathy (Amalric and Biau, 1967; Jain *et al.*, 1967; Okun *et al.*, 1971).

The rationale for the amelioration brought about by this more widespread use of light coagulation seems to lie in the demonstration by Wise (1956) that retinal cells are apt to elaborate a vasoformative stimulus in areas with hypoxia (see p. 14). Focal hypoxia had already been thought to be a significant factor in the pathogenesis of diabetic retinopathy for some years (Ashton, 1953).

On the other hand, no such factor leading to the appearance of new vessels and to the subsequent formation of fibrous tissue is generated in necrotic areas. Hence the advantages derived from transforming all areas where capillary closure or a diminished perfusion exists into biologically inert scars. Furthermore, the fact that an induced descending optic atrophy, as indicated by pallor of the disc and an attenuation of the arterioles, occurs several months or years after extensive coagulation cannot be without effect, as it tends to cause a regression of the epipapillary, papillovitreal and peripapillary neovascular fans.

ARMAMENTARIUM

Photocoagulation was first conducted with the polychromatic light delivered by the xenon-arc lamp. The ruby laser, which is a source of monochromatic light at 6943 Å, has known some measure of popularity, in spite of the fact that the red color of the light precludes its absorption by the retinal vasculature (Beetham *et al.*, 1970).

In addition to the advantage of high spatial and temporal coherence — namely, of the extremely well collimated character of the light — found in lasers generally, the argon laser has brought to the treatment of diabetic retinopathy that of high continuous-wave power (L'Esperance, 1968; L'Esperance *et al.*, 1969; Zweng *et al.*, 1969, 1971; Little *et al.*, 1970). Because of the 70 % absorption by hemoglobin of its predominant wavelengths (4880 Å and 5145 Å) which are in the blue-green spectral region, the argon laser can be applied to the destruction of undesired vessels. It must also be emphasized that though all radiation between 4000 Å and 12000 Å is absorbed to some extent by the pigment epithelium, peak absorption occurs on a wavelength of about 5000 Å. Moreover, the argon laser beam is well transmitted by the eye media.

The utilization of a biomicroscopic delivery system to transport the beam from its source to the eye has several distinct advantages:

1. Both the target area and the surrounding retina can be viewed stereoscopically with varying magnification through a three-mirror contact lens or a macular contact lens.

2. The system provides a large field of view with

excellent background illumination; it neutralizes the patient's refractive error.

3. The size of the beam on the fundus can be adjusted from 50 to 1000 μ, that is from 10′ to 3°20′ approximately.

4. Since the inspection and photocoagulation optical systems are the same, the beam can be brought to sharp focus by simply manipulating the slit-lamp until the target structure is clearly seen.

5. The aiming light on the retina, which is the attenuated laser beam itself, corresponds to the impact diameter of the treating beam; it has a moderate mobility that allows photocoagulation to be performed with some versatility.

The power output into the eye is monitored and can be regulated very gradually up to 1500 mW, which is an important asset in quantitative photocoagulation. Besides, the length of each burst of light can be preset by a precise shutter mechanism from 0.1 second to 1 second, or can be controlled manually as a continuous wave to create the desired effect.

Ham *et al.* (1958) have shown in the rabbit that the total energy required to coagulate a given retinal area decreases considerably with the diameter of the lesion and with the exposure time. Calculation of the thermal effect generated in the retina by photocoagulation has similary shown that the use of small spot diameters with short exposure times results in increased efficiency and in a lessened risk of damage to the nerve fiber layer (Roulier, 1971) *.

Due to its ability to be absorbed well by hemoglobin and melanin, to the predictability of the tissue response, and to the fact that it can produce a considerable thermal rise in the retina with very little energy, the argon laser instrument represents a significant advance in photocoagulation.

TECHNIQUE

In diabetic retinopathy the technique employed should vary with the form and course of the disease. In an effort to introduce some semblance

---

* Fankhauser *et al.* (1972*b*) maintain that the size of the *thermal* spots on the retina remains approximately the same for both the xenon-arc and the argon laser light sources even if the *optical* spots are of a different size. If the exposure time is sufficiently brief and the treated lesion is not in contact with the pigment epithelium this obviously cannot hold true.

of order into what has become a random assortment of different procedures, I once decided to distinguish between three separate therapeutic modalities (Urrets-Zavalía, 1973).

1. There is first what may well be called *focal, precision, target* or *pinpoint bombing,* which is highly selective, must be carried out with great accuracy, and aims at the suppression of vascular abnormalities. By destroying some of the extramacular areas of capillary closure that have been revealed by angiography, it may also be used to reduce the hypoxic stimulus to neovascularization.

2. Secondly, there is what has been termed *systematic, modal* or *oriented bombing* for want of a better name, which tends to act indirectly upon the vascular abnormalities and the ensuing changes in the retinal tissue. The coagulations are arranged in conformity with a preconcieved plan based on structural principles, not on the distribution of lesions. On technical grounds, there is reason to mention four different methods:

a) In one, a great many small photocoagulations of medium intensity are disposed in two almost uninterrupted rows on both sides of all primary and secondary, and of most tertiary retinal veins

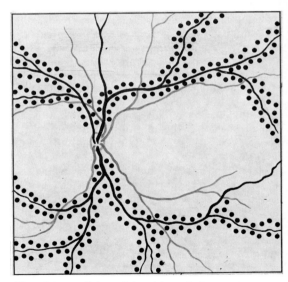

FIG. 8-1. — Oriented bombing of the paravenous, or radial variety.

(Riaskoff, 1972). The coagulation marks extend from the edge of the disc to the equator (Figs. 8-1 and 8-2). The theoretical foundation for this technique lies in the fact that by obliterating a number of the capillaries and postcapillaries that run di-

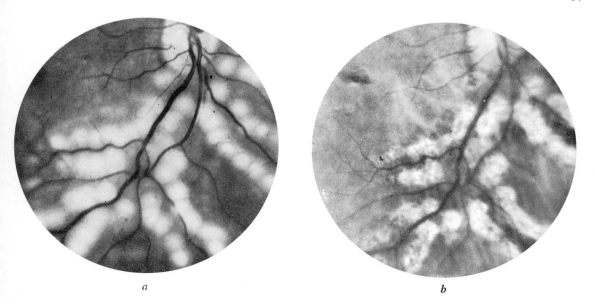

a   *b*

Fig. 8-2. — *a*) An early case of exudative retinopathy one day following argon laser photocoagulation of the paravenous variety (200 µ spot size). *b*) Same area as shown in *a*, 12 months after photocoagulation.

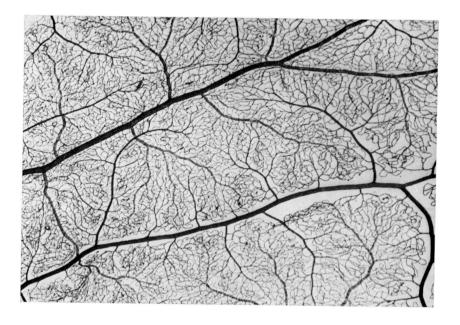

Fig. 8-3. — Human retinal digest preparation showing venules and postcapillaries running directly into a parent vein (larger of the two trunks). Note the capillary-free zone about the arteriole (smaller of the two trunks). (Courtesy Dr. D. Toussaint.)

rectly into the veins one may lessen the engorgement and tortuosity of the veins (Fig. 8-3). This in turn reduces the risk of intravitreal hemorrhage, seals some of the vascular leaks and closes up the source of intraretinal edema, particularly at the macula. In my opinion, it is advisable to spare the arteries, as one does not want to impair the preexisting ischemia by further reducing the blood flow to the retina *. It is the contention of Schiffer and Bonnet (1974) that by occluding shunt vessels at their shedding point in the adjoining veins, this paravenous approach causes the blood flow to pass through the areas of capillary closure under the influence of the head pressure in the parent arterioles (Fig. 8-4).

remains open toward the disc (Rubinstein and Myska, 1972). This technique is indicated whenever the central changes are gross or so close to the fovea that a direct approach would be likely to damage foveal function (Fig. 8-5).

c) In a further method, 200 to 300 photocoagulations of 3° or less are placed in a more or less regular pattern all over the posterior fundus, reaching as far as 4-5 papillary diameters from the disc (Figs 8-6 and 8-7). A bridge of intact retina must be left between each coagulation and the next. No coagulations are placed over the macular or the papillomacular region, and the main vascular arcades are avoided. The purpose of this is

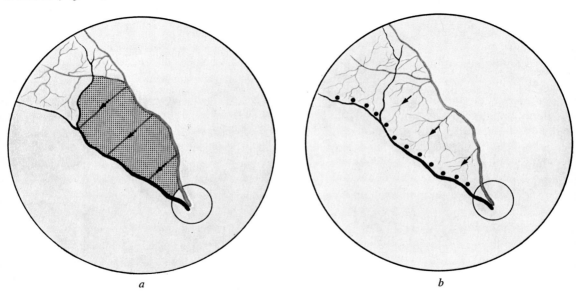

a   *b*

FIG. 8-4. — *a*) Schematic representation of a large area of capillary closure located between an artery and a vein. A number of shunt vessels traverse the area of capillary closure. *b*) By placing an almost uninterrupted row of coagulations along the vein upper margin, the shunt vessels are obliterated at their shedding point and the blood flow is redirected into the areas of nonperfusion. (After SCHIFFER and BONNET, 1974.)

b) In a second method, a perimacular or paramacular approach is practiced, in that a limited number of coagulations are arranged in a horseshoe pattern that surrounds the macula temporally and

---

* The view of Garner and Ashton (1972) that a reduced ophthalmic artery flow with an arteriolar insufficiency within the retina itself must play a significant role in the evolution of the disease is in conflict with the observation by Gay and Rosenbaum (1966) that a lowered pressure in the central retinal artery tends to retard the progression of the retinopathy even in the nonhypertensive patient.

to decrease the cell population in the less critical areas. By reducing the number of retinal elements not vital for good central vision the retina that remains viable becomes better nourished. Under such conditions there should be a decreased metabolic activity, an improved oxygen supply to the surviving tissue and a weakened stimulus to neovascularization (Meyer-Schwickerath and Schott, 1968; Beetham *et al.*, 1969; Wessing, 1972; Wessing and Vogel, 1973).

Visual field defects in patients who have been treated as described are different when assessed

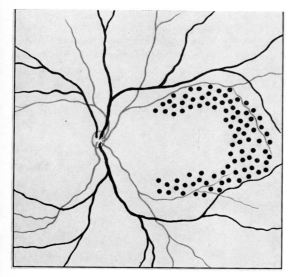

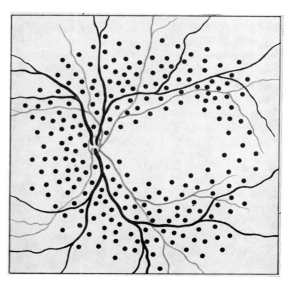

FIG. 8-5. — Distribution of photocoagulation marks in a horseshoe pattern that surrounds the macula temporally.

FIG. 8-6. — Disseminated photocoagulations at the posterior pole. Only the macula, the papillomacular area and the major vascular arcades are spared.

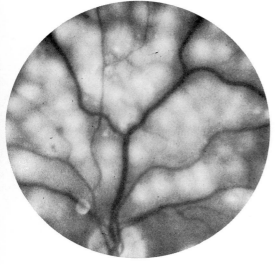

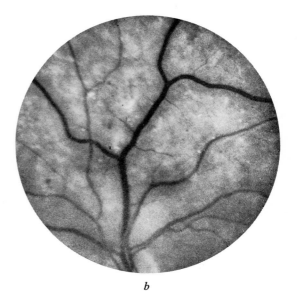

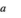 *a*

b

FIG. 8-7. — *a*) Preproliferative diabetic retinopathy one day after disseminated argon laser photocoagulation of the posterior fundus (500 μ spot size). There is a moderate vitreous haze. *b*) Same area as shown in *a*, showing diffuse scarring and clear vitreous two months following photocoagulation.

subjectively and when studied objectively by field plotting. Central changes can of course be detected in every case and appear as discrete scotomas corresponding to the photocoagulation marks. Conduction (nerve fiber bundle) wedge defects are absent unless heavy applications were made in the immediate peripapillary area. Only very rarely, however, do the patients complain of scotomas. This is partly due to the fact that the individual defects are minute, even though multitudinous, and partly to the previous existence of foci of capillary occlusion which had already caused isolated scotomas, as shown by Roth (1969) in the central fields of diabetic patients with and without retinopathy. These defects are merely enlarged by photocoagulation, which does not add much to the patient's disability.

d) Another method consists in carrying out a disseminated coagulation of the peripheral retina, from the equator anteriorly to an imaginary circle that lies some 4-5 papillary diameters from the disc. Several hundred applications of either xenon-arc or laser energy are used, the applications being ordinarily 3° in size; the coagulations must be tangent to each other or no more than one lesion diameter apart (Figs. 8-8 and 8-9). As in the case of the preceding method, therapy is not directed here to any specific abnormality; it aims at the obliteration of a large portion of the retinal surface, Its ultimate goal is to alter the course of the disease, if possible at an early stage, by drastically diminishing the overall circulatory requirements of the retina. Through the widespread destruction of

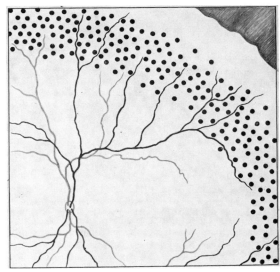

FIG. 8-8. — Retroequatorial photocoagulation. The coagulations are tangent to each other or no more than one disc diameter apart.

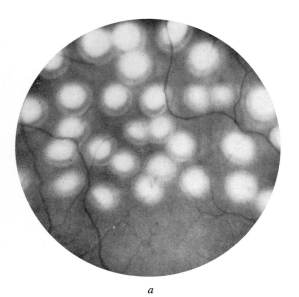

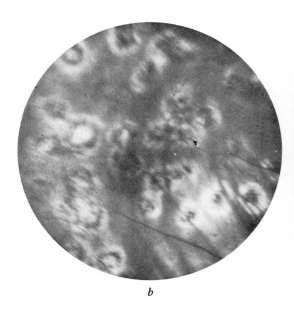

a   *b*

FIG. 8-9. — *a*) Disseminated argon laser photocoagulation of the peripheral retina in an eye with proliferative diabetic retinopathy of the papillovitreal type (1,000 μ spot size). *b*) Same eye, 11 months afterward.

a relatively silent belt area, a certain degree of optic atrophy is induced, which leads to the regression of the neovascularization extending from the disc. Also, as it breaks down the barrier represented by the pigment epithelium, it may be that new pathways of metabolic exchange are established (Peyman *et al.*, 1971).

3. The third form of therapy, which must be regarded as a last-ditch approach to be reserved for those patients with a vasoactivity so great that visual loss through severe intravitreal hemorrhage seems imminent, should be designated as *scatter photocoagulation, multiple peripheral ablative photocoagulation, saturation bombing,* or even *panretinal photocoagulation* (Little, 1973*a;* Urrets-Zavalía, 1973; Zweng, 1973). It affects almost the whole retina from the equator backward, and respects only the disc, the macula, the papillomacular region, and the primary and secondary vascular trunks. Given the amount of coagulation needed, this sort of bombing should be performed ideally with the argon laser system in order to reduce the sum total of energy administered to the eye. All four quadrants are treated in two or three sessions with a 500 to 1000 μ spot. Therefore, it is not unusual to apply 2000 impacts before completing the 360° treatment.

The consequences of this procedure on vision are not as dramatic as may be imagined, which is understandable if one bears in mind that in advanced open-angle glaucoma, patients with a constriction of the field to within 10° or 15° of fixation do not feel immoderately disturbed.

Only in about 20% of the patients in his series who were submitted to massive photocoagulation of the ablative type Frank (1975) found severe visual field loss, in the form of either a large dense nerve fiber defect or a « gun barrel » constriction of isopters to all but the brightest and largest test.

Using electroretinography to estimate the total retinal area destroyed in massive photocoagulation, Frank concluded that that area amounts to approximately 40 %. This suggests that extensive photocoagulation may alter very considerably both the quantitative aspects of retinal metabolism and retinal hemodynamics.

Whatever the technique used, it should be noted that improvement of vision is not the main goal of treatment, a fact which must repeatedly be brought to the patient's attention. Rather, in the face of progressive retinopathy, *stabilization* is the desired objective. Cessation of bleeding, permanent vitreous clearing and the drying up of an edematous macula do entail a definite functional

gain. As Spalter (1971) has put it, improvement in acuity in addition to stabilization is an agreeable dividend but not a prime consideration.

Now, let us refer in detail to the forms of treatment particularly suited to the different types of diabetic retinopathy that have been dealt with previously.

I. — NONPROLIFERATIVE OR SIMPLE DIABETIC RETINOPATHY

1° In the predominantly exudative form the treatment should effect an obliteration of the microaneurysms — particularly those with a yellowish halo — and intraretinal abnormal capillaries located in the immediate vicinity of the large waxy deposits or in the center of the circinate complexes which develop in the macula or are lateral to it. *A priori* reasoning suggests that closure of the vascular leakage sites should prevent further retinal edema, allow a resorption of the hard exudates and reduce visual morbidity. Such a theoretical consideration has been confirmed by clinical results (Spalter, 1971, 1972; Bonnet and Pingault, 1971; Bonnet, 1972).

Because of its efficacy in destroying microaneurysms and shunt vessels the xenon-arc coagulator may be used to this end, but only as long as the applications remain at a minimal distance of one-half to one disc diameter from the fovea (Fig. 8-10). An added difficulty with the xenon-arc apparatus is the smallness of the observation field; this may cause the operator to lose his bearings as he comes near the macula, where there are few blood vessels that can be used as a guide.

The argon laser photocoagulator knows no such limitations and therefore is preferable to treat exudative maculopathy (Figs. 8-11 and 8-12). In general, only the 50 and 100 μ spot sizes are used with 200 to 300 mW power at 0.1 and 0.2 seconds. As the retinal tissue is usually edematous in the neighborhood of the fovea, a considerable amount of energy is absorbed by the protein in the extracellular fluid before the light beam reaches the pigment epithelium. The coagulations must be moderately heavy to produce thrombosis and permanent occlusion of the leaking vessels; a higher intensity should be used if the effect is poor.

It has been my experience that one must not come closer than 100 μ from the fovea; this is due less to the very tiny scotoma which is produced than to the cicatricial damage to the adjacent retina. In order to spare a fovea which may be ob-

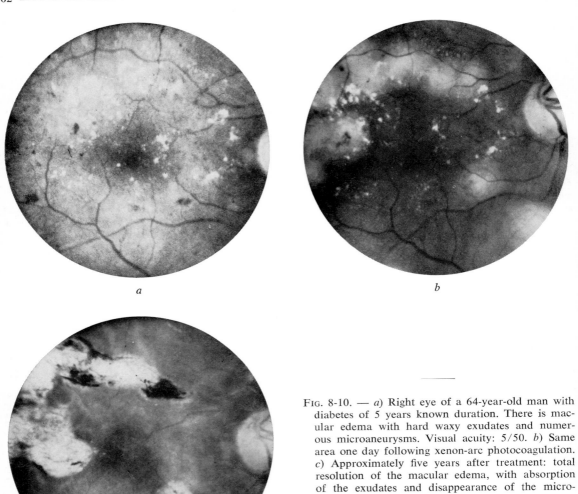

a

b

c

Fig. 8-10. — *a*) Right eye of a 64-year-old man with diabetes of 5 years known duration. There is macular edema with hard waxy exudates and numerous microaneurysms. Visual acuity: 5/50. *b*) Same area one day following xenon-arc photocoagulation. *c*) Approximately five years after treatment: total resolution of the macular edema, with absorption of the exudates and disappearance of the microaneurysms. Visual acuity: 5/10.

scured by the existing edema or hard exudates, I have found it expedient to localize it by instructing the patient to look at the star of the Visuscope. This is still possible with a visual acuity of 5/50 or less. The examiner observes the point of the fundus on which the star is projected and correlates its position to that of a detectable landmark.

Remission is indicated by a diminished venous congestion and a resorption of macular edema; aneurysms and exudates and even some vascular lesions that have not been subjected to direct coagulation tend to disappear at a later date. In general

the early effects of treatment cannot be observed for several weeks, and the full effect for several months. The greater the influence of ageing, of high blood pressure or the metabolic disturbance itself on the retinal vascular bed, the longer it will take for a favorable response to appear. Thus, in those over 60 years of age, progressive improvement can still be detected after three or four years. Drying up of the macula will result in improved acuity only when the treatment is carried out early enough. If microcystoid changes are shown to be present by contact lens examination, the prognosis is poor as these are apt to persist indefinitely; individual cysts may even merge into a larger cavity or proceed to give rise to a macular hole, so that central vision continues to deteriorate. Resorption of fatty exudates usually produces only a limited visual amelioration at best, since neuronal damage has already set in. Nevertheless, it is erroneous to say that the treatment is of little or no avail, for if the disease is brought to a standstill further visual decline will be prevented.

The macular pucker syndrome which results from peripheral photocoagulation is seldom seen

2° ***In the hemorrhagic type*** of diabetic retinopathy the importance of high-resolution fluorescein angiography as an adjunct to photocoagulation cannot be overemphasized. For practical purposes, the following therapeutic plan may be recommended:

Target bombing should be used to destroy microaneurysms which appear as leaking points in the angiogram, intraretinal dilated capillaries, and areas of avascularity (Fig. 8-14).

Bombing oriented along dilated and irregular veins, particularly in those segments where their

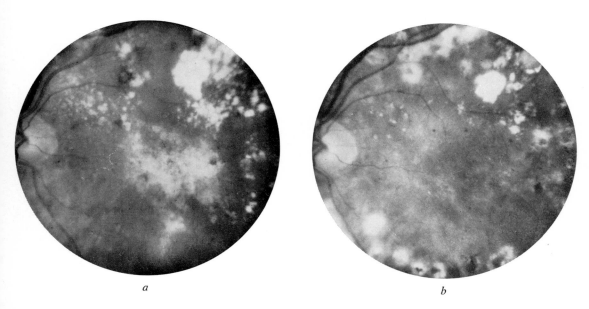

a *b*

Fɪɢ. 8-11. — *a*) Right fundus of a 68-year-old man with diabetes of 17 years duration showing edema of central retina, gross waxy exudates and multiples microaneurysms. Visual acuity: 1/15. *b*) Eighteen months after argon laser photocoagulation there is a marked decrease in the amount of exudate, total resolution of the edema and disappearance of visible angiopathy. Visual acuity: 5/15.

in diabetic retinopathy. However, the development of a fibrous epiretinal membrane over the whole macular area with subsequent shrinkage and severe morphological distortion may be observed occasionally (Fig. 8-13). This so-called *surface-wrinkling retinopathy* comes from the administration of an excessive amout of radiation to the delicate macular and papillomacular structures, which should always be approached with caution but especially so in cases with diffuse edema at the posterior pole, and in those where a massive effusion becomes apparent in the late phases of fluorescein angiography.

wall retains the fluorescent dye, must start at the disc and proceed to the equator; reduplicated venous segments and venous coils or loops should also be treated in this way (Fig. 8-15). Disseminated bombing of the extramacular retina, in the intervals between the larger vessels, or peripheral bombing at or near the equator is also necessary (Fig. 8-16).

Large preretinal hemorrhages of the swallow's nest and the oval varieties should be left alone, particularly if located near the macula, as the increased absorption of light by blood will heat the internal limiting membrane and the vitreous

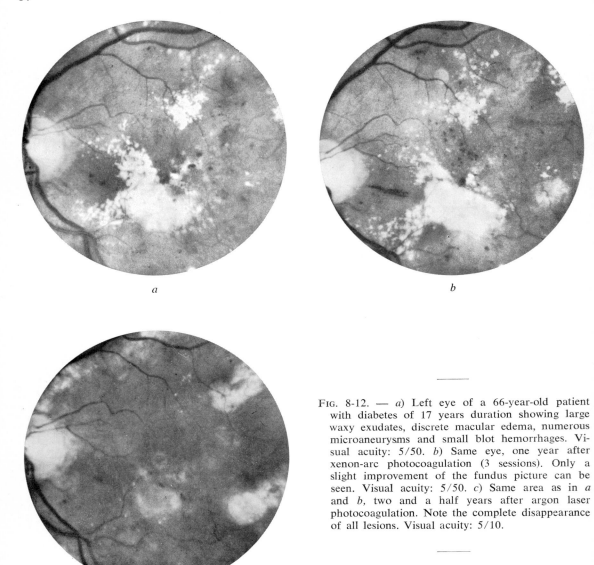

a

b

c

FIG. 8-12. — *a*) Left eye of a 66-year-old patient with diabetes of 17 years duration showing large waxy exudates, discrete macular edema, numerous microaneurysms and small blot hemorrhages. Visual acuity: 5/50. *b*) Same eye, one year after xenon-arc photocoagulation (3 sessions). Only a slight improvement of the fundus picture can be seen. Visual acuity: 5/50. *c*) Same area as in *a* and *b*, two and a half years after argon laser photocoagulation. Note the complete disappearance of all lesions. Visual acuity: 5/10.

cortex *. Only the site of origin of such a hemorrhage should be treated directly (Figs. 8-17

and 8-18). In some instances the source of the hemorrhage is several disc diameters away from the pool of blood; a small coagulum still adherent to a dilated vein may permit identification of the leaking point (Okun *et al.*, 1971). The placement of coagulations over the blood clot itself is permissible in the case of the smaller preretinal hemorrhages, which will then resorb and be replaced by an atrophic scar.

*It should be noted that most of the so-called pre-retinal or subhyaloid hemorrhages are situated between the nerve fiber layer and the internal limiting membrane, and that only after rupture of this membrane does the blood spread under the outer vitreous face or pour into the vitreous cavity.

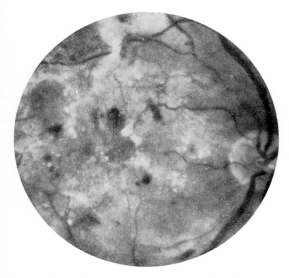

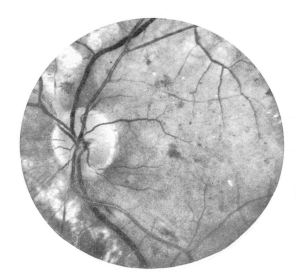

FIG. 8-13. — Same eye as shown in Fig. 3-3 (page 21), six months following moderately heavy argon laser photocoagulation. Scarring is not very marked but an epiretinal membrane has developed over the macular area. Visual acuity: 1/30.

FIG. 8-14. — Same eye as shown in Fig. 3-7 (page 24), one and a half years after argon laser photocoagulation (target and disseminated posterior bombing). There is almost complete disappearance of the retinal hemorrhages; no hard exudates are left. Note pallor of the optic disc and decreased distension of the veins with regularization in caliber. Visual acuity: 5/7.5.

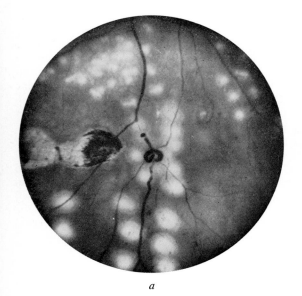

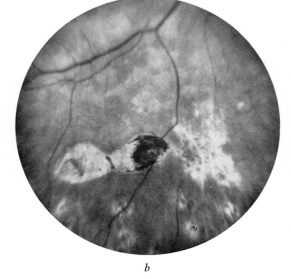

a   *b*

FIG. 8-15. — *a*) Right fundus of a 47-year-old woman with diabetes of 27 years duration. There is an omega-like loop on a vein that has been bleeding repeatedly; note old photocoagulation scar. This protograph was taken ten minutes after argon laser treatment. *b*) At the end of one year the vascular abnormality has been replaced by a new photocoagulation scar; note the marked decrease in the caliber of the veins.

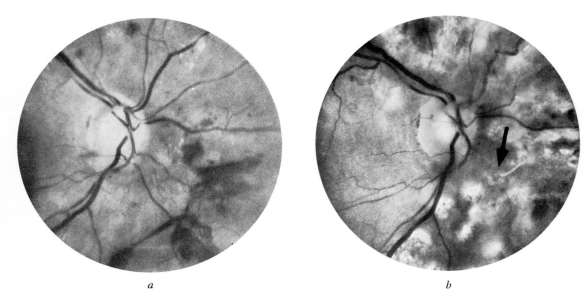

a   *b*

FIG. 8-16. — *a*) Right eye of a 64-year-old woman with diabetes of 12 years known duration. Multiple, medium-sized hemorrhages are scattered over the posterior fundus. *b*) Two years after argon laser saturation bombing of the posterior pole only a few isolated hemorrhages remain. Note complete occlusion of a venule nasally to the disc (arrow).

II. — PROLIFERATIVE
OR MALIGNANT DIABETIC RETINOPATHY

In the treatment of the malignant type of diabetic retinopathy, one should consider separately the neovascularization which develops on the retinal surface, the neovascularization on the optic nerve-head, and that which extends into the vitreous space and is either bare or enmeshed in a variable amount of glial tissue (L'Esperance, 1969, 1973; Dobree, 1970; Taylor, 1970; Little and Zweng, 1971; Patz, 1972; Zweng *et al.*, 1972; Dobree and Taylor, 1973).

1° Surface retinal neovascularization. —
When the neovascularization afflicts areas other than the disc and develops in the plane of the retina, the first coagulations should be confined to the new vessels themselves and the surrounding retina. All of the irregular tufts arising from dilated veins that are still on or close to the retinal surface, as well as the cartwheel-like neovascular formations that extend over the internal limiting membrane are amenable to treatment with either the xenon-arc or the argon laser photocoagulator (Figs. 8-19 and 8-20). Fairly confluent 1.5° to 3°

(500 to 1000 μ.) coagulations should cover the lesions and extend a half disc diameter beyond them in all directions to prevent recurrences (Fig. 8-21). Although it is not necessary to create a dead-white plaque, the intensity must be sufficient to produce retinal necrosis, leaving behind a yellowish, atrophic scar and not merely a slate-colored one. Immediate obliteration of the blood column in all the affected vessels is desirable (Dobree and Taylor, 1968). In this, as in a number of other different situations, overbombing (or the obliteration of a target with more force than required) is inadvisable as it would be liable to make a bad situation worse.

The treatment canot be confined however to target bombing if the elimination of all potential sources of vitreous hemorrhages and a lessened risk of recurrent neovascularization are to be achieved (Fig. 8-22). Both an oriented bombing along the retinal veins, which are engorged and of an uneven caliber and very often show a number of hairpin or omega-like loops, and some retroequatorial bombing to reduce the metabolic requirements of the retina should be done.

2° Epi- and peripapillary neovascularization. — Early neovascularization that lies flat on the optic nervehead or extends centrifugally over the surrounding retina should be approached directly with the argon laser beam, using a 50 μ spot size, a power level of about 200 mW and an exposure time of 0.1 to 0.5 second (Figs. 8-23 and 8-24). While the desired endpoint of treatment is the immediate closure of the vessels being coagulated, with interruption of blood flow, this may occur only after several weeks.

It must be noted that, with the xenon-arc instrument, photocoagulation adjacent to the disc occasionally results in atrophy of the new vessels on its surface and even of vessels extending into elevated proliferative tufts (Figs 8-25 and 8-26).

3° Papillovitreal neovascularization. — Neovascular formations extending from the disc anteriorly should also be treated with the argon laser photocoagulator (Figs. 8-27, 8-28 and 8-29). If the new vessels are few and unaccompanied by visible connective tissue they may be picked off

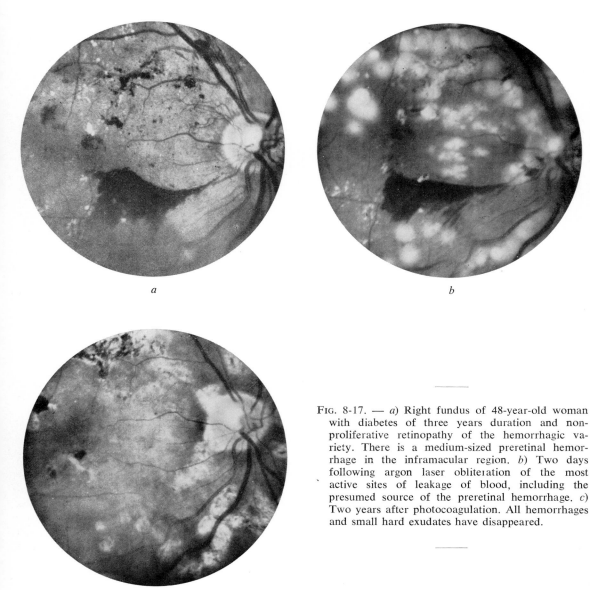

a

b

c

FIG. 8-17. — *a*) Right fundus of 48-year-old woman with diabetes of three years duration and nonproliferative retinopathy of the hemorrhagic variety. There is a medium-sized preretinal hemorrhage in the inframacular region. *b*) Two days following argon laser obliteration of the most active sites of leakage of blood, including the presumed source of the preretinal hemorrhage. *c*) Two years after photocoagulation. All hemorrhages and small hard exudates have disappeared.

one by one with the 50 μ spot. If the neovascularization is heavy, in the form of a florid, seafan-shaped frond, and is supported by cloud condensation of fibrous tissue, every effort should be made to identify the arterial feeders to the frond in high-resolution enlargements made from the early fluorescein photographs (Figs. 8-30 and 8-31). Such arterial feeders can be made visible in about one third of all cases.

In those cases where the feeder or afferent vessels have been located, multiple applications of the laser beam are delivered until they become attenuated or occluded, or until the blood column

lation of the collector channels from a neovascular frond without closing the feeders first is dangerous. The objective of this technique is the avoidance of venous engorgement with subsequent hemorrhage. As the apparent obliteration seen clinically during and immediately following photocoagulation may only represent a transitory spasm, it is advisable to have the patient return in a few hours for examination. If some of the treated vessels are now patent, additional photocoagulation is applied. When recanalization occurs at a later date, retreatment may convert an initial failure into a success.

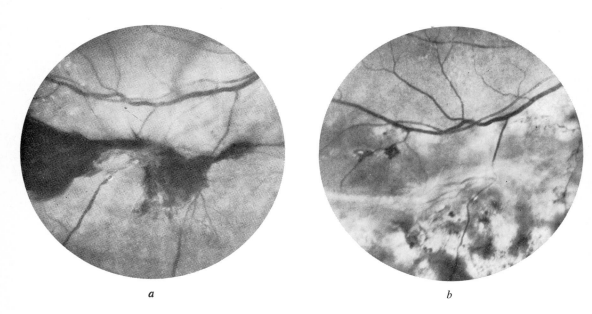

a   *b*

FIG. 8-18. — *a*) Right eye of a 56-year-old woman with diabetes of 15 years duration. Note a large boat-shaped preretinal hemorrhage located below the inferotemporal arcade. *b*) Five years after heavy xenon-arc photocoagulation of the affected area. The retina has become sclerosed and is covered in part by a thin fibrous membrane.

fragments. As soon as the neovascular frond becomes ischemic, it is coagulated in turn. Following this, the larger outflow vessels can be attacked. In every instance the diameter of the treating beam should be at least one and a half times the vessel width. When the angiogram has not definitely identified the feeders, one should remember that the narrower vessels are more likely to be on the feeder side of the tuft and the larger vessels on the drainage side. In any event, stress must be laid on the fact that coagu-

It is the contention of Fankhauser *et al.* (1972*a* and *b*) that photocoagulation with the argon laser offers no advantages over the coagulation conducted with their optical attachement to the Zeiss xenon-arc instrument for use with the Haag-Streit slit-lamp. Not having had any experience with that device, I am in no position to pass judgement upon the validity of their claim.

When the new vessels are ensconced in a matrix of connective tissue, only a coagulation of the feeder vessels should be attempted — or coagulation of those vessels that have bled recently — inasmuch as treatment of the sheets and strands themselves would result in retraction, in an extension of the fibroglial reaction, or both. Although the afferent vessels in the fibrotic bands are difficult to coagulate, because the collagen in the bands reflects and disperses the light, some very good results may be obtained if that technique is used (Figs. 8-32 and 8-33).

While very easy to photocoagulate because of their deep red color, the berry-like clumps of vascular tissue which appear sometimes on the disc must be hit with caution, as they may be the starting point of a profuse hemorrhage.

With a view to minimizing the problem of recurrent neovascularization by acting indirectly on the intravitreal networks, coagulation of the networks themselves should always be supplemented with a more or less extensive photocoagulation of the extramacular retina. This may be carried out at once or after a few weeks. It seems indeed that widespread photocoagulation — or photocoagulation applied only to distant areas of the retina — may bring about a regression of optic disc neo-

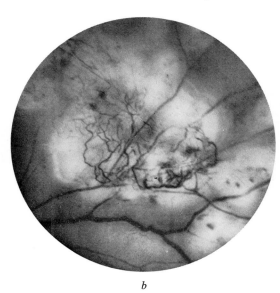

a

b

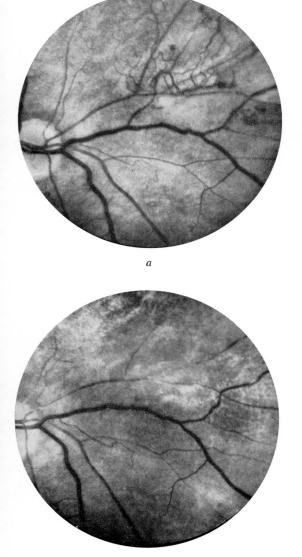

FIG. 8-19. — *a*) Left fundus of a 55-year-old man with diabetes of 12 years duration. There is a large fan of surface neovascularization spreading over the superonasal quadrant. *b*) One day following xenon-arc photocoagulation. *c*) Seven years after treatment. Elimination of all visible new vessels has been accomplished, with replacement by only mild cicatricial changes.

c

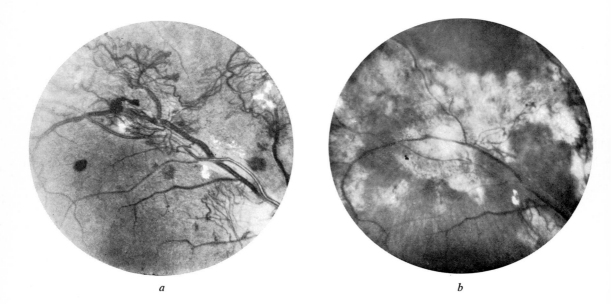

FIG. 8-20. — *a*) Right eye of a 22-year-old man with diabetes of 15 years known duration and florid proliferative retinopathy. Note the extensive fan of neovascularization originating from superotemporal veins. *b*) Appearance of the same area three years after argon laser photocoagulation. No new vessels remain.

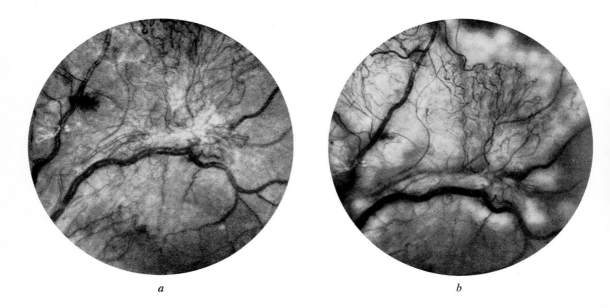

FIG. 8-21. — *a*) Right eye of a 48-year-old man with diabetes of ten years duration and advanced proliferative retinopathy. One sees of profuse spider-web-like network of surface neovascularization in the superonasal quadrant. *b*) The appearance one day after argon laser photocoagulation which covers the lesions and extends a half disc diameter into the surrounding retina.

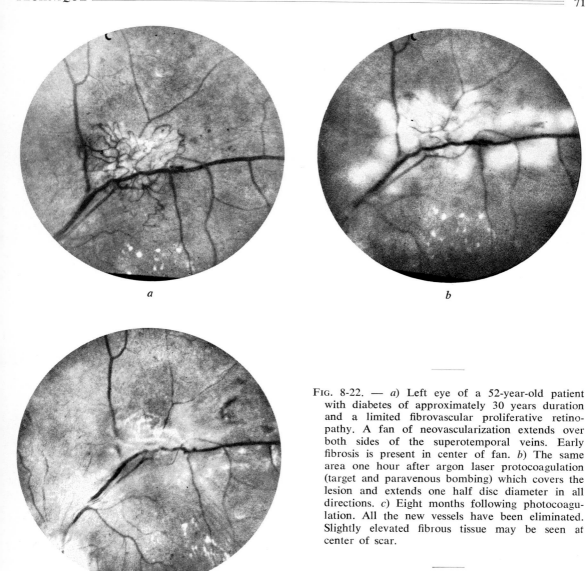

FIG. 8-22. — *a*) Left eye of a 52-year-old patient with diabetes of approximately 30 years duration and a limited fibrovascular proliferative retinopathy. A fan of neovascularization extends over both sides of the superotemporal veins. Early fibrosis is present in center of fan. *b*) The same area one hour after argon laser protocoagulation (target and paravenous bombing) which covers the lesion and extends one half disc diameter in all directions. *c*) Eight months following photocoagulation. All the new vessels have been eliminated. Slightly elevated fibrous tissue may be seen at center of scar.

vascularization. This is dependent upon the extent of the chorioretinal burns, which should then involve a minimum of 20 % of the total retinal area, and upon the type of disc neovascularization: the early category in which regression occurs is that in which the new vessels are flat — or nearly so — and devoid of visible fibrous sheathing (Taylor, 1970). Saturation bombing may bring about stabilization even after some connective tissue

develops around the naked vessels, although no actual regression may occur. Pan-retinal or saturation bombing must be considered as an initial procedure when the feeder vessels cannot be identified, or when a prepapillary frond is unusually large and should ideally be reduced in size. James and l'Esperance (1974) also use this technique as a first step for fronds with too much fibrous tissue to allow the direct treatment approach, and

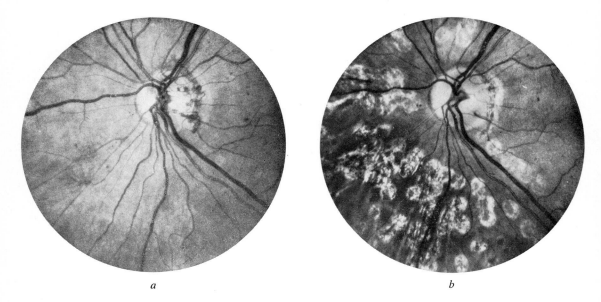

a   *b*

FIG. 8-23. — *a*) Left eye of a 45-year-old patient with diabetes of 12 years duration and early proliferative retinopathy of the epipapillary type. *b*) Complete regression of epipapillary new vessels two and a half years after argon laser photocoagulation (target bombing directed at all neovascular tufts, plus pan-retinal saturation bombing).

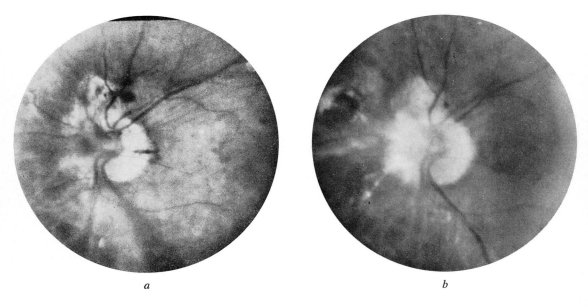

a   *b*

FIG. 8-24. — *a*) Left fundus of a 72-year-old woman with diabetes of 24 years duration. Epipapillary neovascularization is seen with a slight fibrotic component. There have been several bleeding episodes and the vitreous is hazy. *b*) Eighteen months after argon laser treatment. All new vessels have been replaced by photocoagulation scars, there is pallor of the disc, and the vitreous is clear.

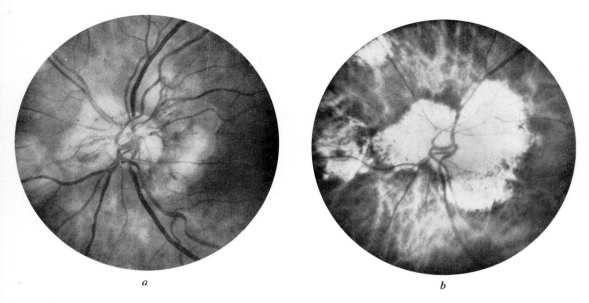

a
b

Fɪɢ. 8-25. — *a*) Left fundus of a 42-year-old man with diabetes of 20 years duration. Photograph taken one day following xenon-arc treatment of an early neovascular frond that lies flat on the optic nervehead and extends centrifugally over the surrounding retina. Visual acuity: 5/5. *b*) After an interval of eight years there are no new vessels visible. In spite of the markedly atrophic character of the resulting scar, the visual acuity is still 5/5.

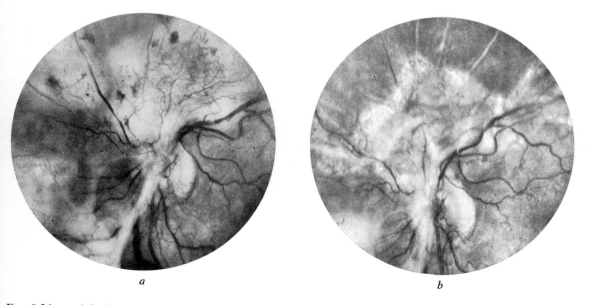

a
b

Fɪɢ. 8-26. — *a*) Left eye of a 63-year-old man with diabetes of 21 years duration and proliferative retinopathy with advanced fibrovascular membrane formation. The photograph was taken ten minutes after extensive xenon-arc photocoagulation. *b*) Four years after treatment, the same eye shows marked regression of all lesions and arrest of the disease process.

URRETS-ZAVALIA.

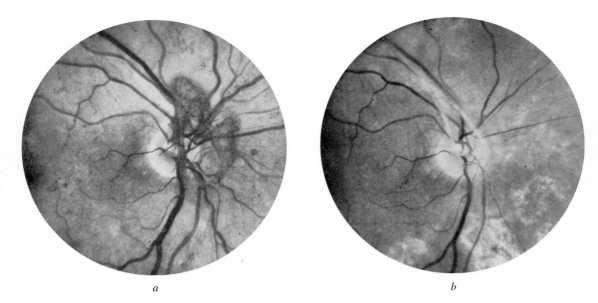

a   *b*

FIG. 8-27. — *a*) Right eye of a 67-year-old woman with diabetes of unknown duration and proliferative retinopathy of the papillovitreal type. No feeder vessels could be identified in the early stages of fluorescein
fundus photography. *b*) The same eye, 18 months after heavy argon laser photocoagulation (direct bombing
of the new vessels at and near the disc plus pan-retinal bombing). There is complete disappearance of the
lesions, which have been replaced by two narrow fibrotic bands.

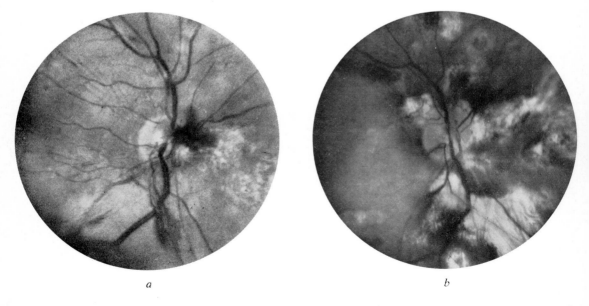

a   *b*

FIG. 8-28. — *a*) Right fundus of a 51-year-old man with diabetes of 18 years duration. Two neovascular
proliferative tufts are advancing from the disc into the vitreous chamber. On the nasal side of disc is
an old photocoagulation scar. The vitreous is moderately hazy. *b*) Twenty months after argon laser photocoagulation there are no new vessels left and the vitreous is clear.

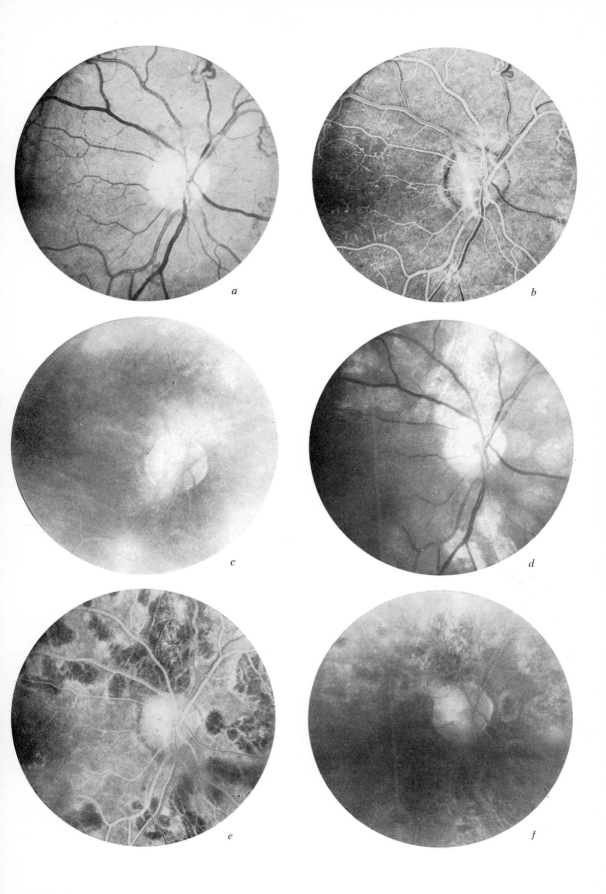

in those cases when vitreous traction around the optic nerve would make photocoagulation hazardous. On the basis of what has been said above and of the accumulated experience with vitrectomy, I am of the opinion that the eyes in these last categories no longer fall within the province of photocoagulation but should rather be treated by vitrectomy.

4° *Retinovitreal neovascularization.* — Any retinal proliferation extending into the vitreous should be treated by placing a number of rather intense photocoagulations around its base (Fig. 8-34). In most cases this will cause atrophy of the neovascular component in the proliferative growth. In the case of foci of tenuous neovascularization which are often encountered in the posterior vitreous as webs without visible or clear connections to the underlying retina, durable obliteration can only be achieved with argon laser photocoagulation (Fig. 8-35).

There are eyes in which the feeders to a florid preretinal neovascular network may be identified in the angiogram (Fig. 8-36). Treatment should aim first at the obliteration of these and be directed only afterward at the core of the network and the neighboring retina. The results may not be satisfactory, however, for new zones of neovascularization may appear peripheral to the treated one. For the most part the mulberry-like, oval or round bundles of dense fibrovascular tissue which develop in the posterior vitreous just over the retinal surface are amenable to treatment (Fig. 8-37). Still, it sometimes happens that even heavy photocoagulation does not bring about regression, for recanalization occurs and is followed by bleeding.

Once the condition has reached the stage, usually described in superlatives, where extensive glial and fibrous proliferation exists, photocoagulation is often useless because the new vessels have receded spontaneously; it may be inoperative, and even contraindicated as when the masses of

fibrous tissue are so exuberant that they can no longer be approached with any measure of safety. If the detached vitreous is retracted and exerts a strong pull upon a papillovitreal stalk or membrane, no amount or form of light coagulation will protect the patient from the risk of massive hemorrhage or a traction retinal detachment.

INDICATIONS FOR TREATMENT

Photocoagulation is indicated in some combinations of circumstances. Consideration must be given to: (*a*) progression of the condition as revealed by both direct fundus examination and fluorescein angiography, (*b*) the form of the disease, (*c*) the age of the patient, and (*d*) the fasting plasma level of somatotrophin.

Cases with only a few microaneurysms, scattered small hemorrhages and isolated hard exudates are kept under observation. Treatment is recommended in the event that a complicating macular edema with visual impairment (5/15 or worse) develops, particularly when lipoid deposits appear near the fovea in atoll-like formations or large plaques. The disclosure by angiography of a great number of microaneurysms and intraretinal dilated capillaries in an eye where only scant changes had been found before suggests that photocoagulation should be performed immediately. In the young particularly, periodic controls are definitely required because a sudden efflorescence of such abnormalities may occur and a veritable *rubeosis retinae* appear unexpectedly. The presence of such venous changes as pronounced dilatation, beading, and loops is of similar import, as is also the appearance of multiple, extensive retinal hemorrhages or of a large number of soft exudates. Patients with *any degree* of neovascularization either in the plane of the retina or disc or advancing into the vitreous

---

Legend of figure on previous page.

FIG. 8-29. — *a*) The right fundus of a 34-year-old man with diabetes of 23 years duration. Note epi- and peri-papillary neovascular fronds of the naked-vessel variety, isolated foci of surface retinal neovascularization, and one abnormal venous loop at the 12:30 o'clock position. *b*) An early arteriovenous phase angiogram does not permit identification of the afferent vessels, as the whole neovascular system is already filled with dye. *c*) A late phase angiogram shows diffuse leakage into vitreous cavity. *d*) Fourteen months after argon laser photocoagulation treatment (pan-retinal photocoagulation, plus direct bombing of the neovascular frond and abnormal venous loop) there is complete disappearance of all visible lesions. *e*) and *f*) Both early arteriovenous phase and late phase angiograms fail to show any abnormality, apart from the photocoagulation scars.

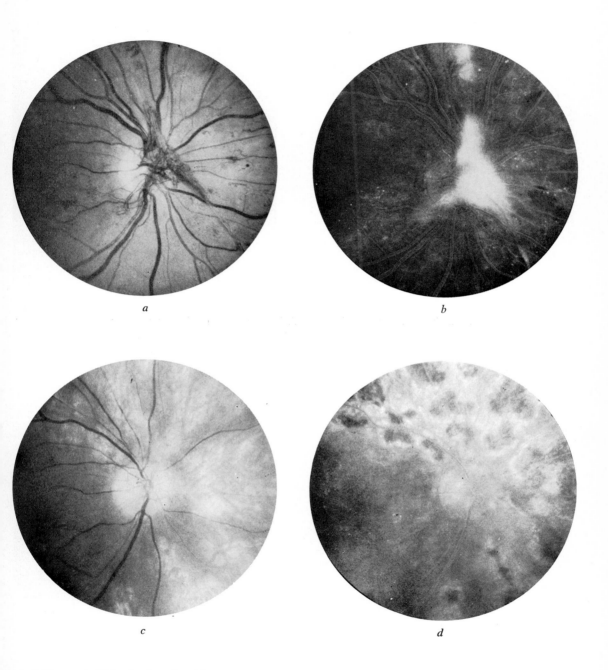

FIG. 8-30. — *a*) Right fundus of a 29-year-old female with known diabetes since the age of three. A dense, closely packed neovascular bundle arises from the optic nervehead. Other, isolated epiretinal new vessels are scattered over the posterior pole. *b*) A late venous phase angiogram shows a profuse leak from the papillovitreal new vessels. *c*) Eighteen months following argon laser bombing of the arterial vessels to the frond; saturation bombing of the retroequatorial retina was also carried out as a supportive measure. All abnormal vessels have disappeared without a trace. Note marked reduction in the caliber of both arteries and veins. *d*) In the late (recirculation) phase angiogram no abnormal channels and no leakage of dye can be seen.

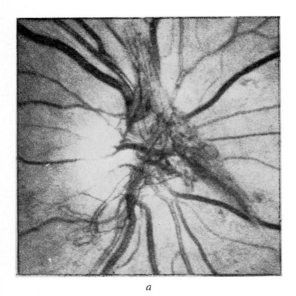 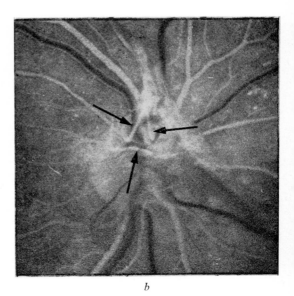

a   *b*

FIG. 8-31. — *a*) Same fundus as shown in Fig. 8-30. A high resolution enlargement from disc and adjoining areas. *b*) Early arterial phase angiogram showing arterial feeders to papillovitreal frond (arrows). The new vessels are still not completely perfused.

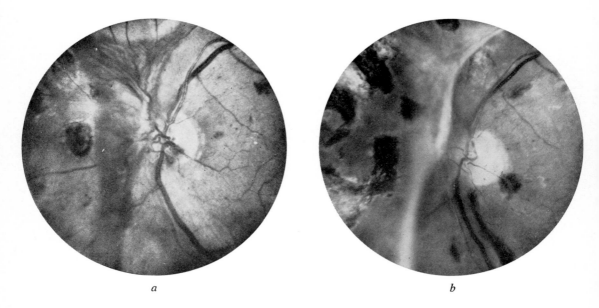

a   *b*

FIG. 8-32. — *a*) Left fundus of a 52-year-old man with diabetes of 19 years duration. A highly elevated fibro-vascular membrane arises from the optic disc. On the nasal side are old photocoagulation scars. *b*) Forty-one months following argon laser obliteration of the afferent vessels there is marked regression of neo-vascular component.

should be treated at once, before the disease reaches the stage where it can only be subjected to other, more complicated forms of therapy (Fig. 8-38).

If there is a highly elevated mean level of serum growth hormone, with wild variations in the 24-hour curve, the prognosis must be guarded as new bleeding episodes and recurrent neovas-cularization may be anticipated in the patients with the hemorrhagic and the early proliferative forms of retinopathy.

The attitude to be assumed toward advanced fibrotic lesions and secondary retinal detachment which can no longer benefit from light coagulation shall be discussed later.

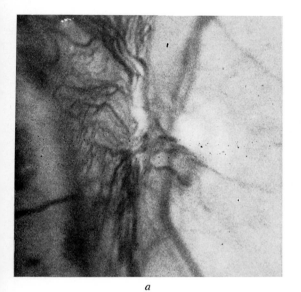

a

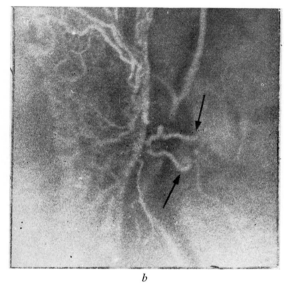

b

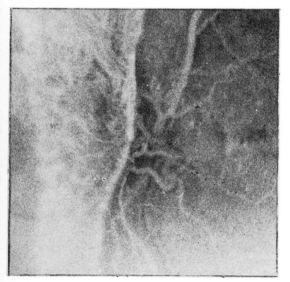

c

FIG. 8-33. — *a*) Same eye as shown in Fig. 8-32. A high resolution enlargement from optic disc and adjoining area. *b*) An arterial phase angiogram permits identification of the afferent vessels to the large papillovitreal fibrovascular band (arrows). *c*) In the arteriovenous phase the dye fills the neovascular web in its entirety; some leakage is already apparent.

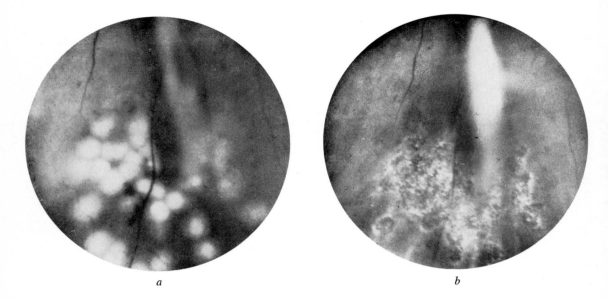

a   *b*

FIG. 8-34. — *a*) Left eye of a 32-year-old woman with known diabetes since the age of 4. A retinovitreal stalk with moderate neovascularization can be seen. (Fundus photograph taken immediately following argon laser treatment.) *b*) One year after photocoagulation there no longer is any discernible vascular component.

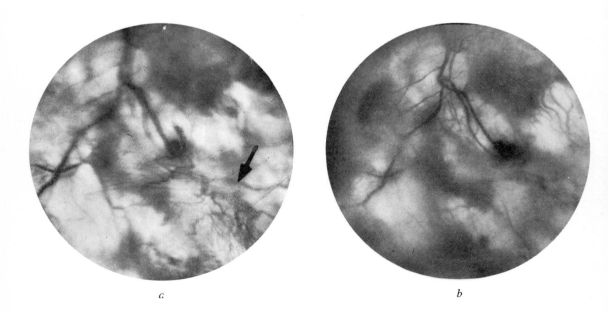

a   *b*

FIG. 8-35. — *a*) Left fundus of a 74-year-old woman with diabetes of 20-odd years duration. After heavy treatment with xenon-arc photocoagulation some intravitreal new vessels which bleed intermittently still persist in lower temporal fundus (arrow). *b*) Three and a half years after argon laser photocoagulation (target bombing) all of the abnormal vessels have disappeared. No further bleeding episodes have occurred.

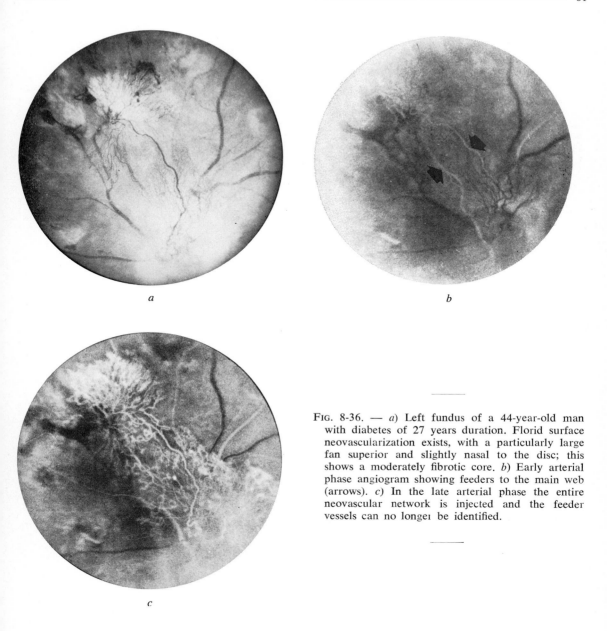

a

b

Fig. 8-36. — *a*) Left fundus of a 44-year-old man with diabetes of 27 years duration. Florid surface neovascularization exists, with a particularly large fan superior and slightly nasal to the disc; this shows a moderately fibrotic core. *b*) Early arterial phase angiogram showing feeders to the main web (arrows). *c*) In the late arterial phase the entire neovascular network is injected and the feeder vessels can no longer be identified.

c

RESULTS

Whenever an adequate intensity has been used, photocoagulation leads to a disappearance of the normal and abnormal retinal capillaries, and of most of the directly treated microaneurysms and new vessels on the retinal surface or extending slightly into the vitreous. This occurs after an interval of several weeks and can always be seen in the angiogram, where a dark area of nonperfusion exists at the place of each cicatricial mark. On the basis of what I have seen in many postoperative angiograms, I disagree with the assertion by Archer *et al.* (1970) that light coagulation has little effect on the number of microaneurysms

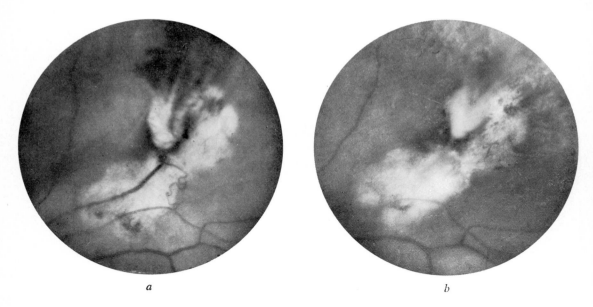

a   *b*

Fig. 8-37. — *a*) Left fundus of a 43-year old woman with diabetes of ten years duration. There was a history of repeated vitreous hemorrhages which could be traced to a dense preretinal bundle of fibrovascular tissue located superiorly. Previous xenon-arc photocoagulation had been ineffectual. *b*) Twenty-six months after argon laser treatment there remains only an avascular fibrous mass and all hemorrhagic activity has ceased.

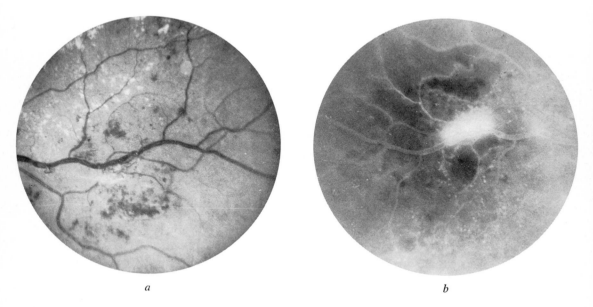

a   *b*

Fig. 8-38. — *a*) Right eye of a 62-year-old man with diabetes of 18 years duration. Direct fundus examination reveals a large cluster of dot hemorrhages, small scattered hard exudates and very early neovascularization which originates from the superotemporal vein. *b*) A recirculation phase fluorescein angiogram shows, in addition to microaneurysms, multiple areas of capillary closure and severe damage to vascular walls, all signs that treatment must be instituted at once.

and on the number and distribution of vascular shunts. The main retinal arteries and veins remain initialy unaffected as a consequence of the protection afforded by their multicoated, considerably thicker walls and by the rapid heat transfer produced by the greater volume of circulating blood. The effect of both the xenon-arc and the argon laser beam is not limited to the retina, however, for at the end of a few months a complete atrophy of the choroidal vasculature also occurs, as shown by the development of yellowish spots surrounded by more or less heavily pigmented rims. In this connection, we must not be misled by the histological and ultrastructural short-term findings of Apple *et al.* (1973) and of Limon *et al.* (1973). If in these studies, respectively, there was no consistent occlusion of the retinal capillaries and of the choriocapillaries after argon laser photocoagulation, this was because the observations were made at the end of only 24 hours. The same be said of the observations of Lerche and Beeger (1972), who found only an infiltration first of granulocytes and then of histiocytes in the hours following ruby laser photocoagulation.

When the neovascularization shows a definite invasive tendency the response is less impressive, even when the argon laser is used. Obliteration of both the new vessels which lie flat on the fundus and those which arise from the disc or retina into the vitreous is considered to have occurred when one of the two following conditions has been met six months after photocoagulation:

a) the neovascularization is no longer visible ophthalmoscopically;

b) perfusion of the treated vessels is angiographically absent or visible only in an attenuated form.

Some control of the neovascularization is thought to have been achieved when a limited glial reinforcement of the new vessels has occurred without additional neovascular growth or rupture, or when fluorescein extravasation from the treated vessels is no longer present in areas of the angiogram where it had been detected before (L'Esperance, 1973).

As decreased leakage from the abnormal vasculature in the directly treated, adjacent, or even remote areas takes place the hemorrhagic activity stops. Occasionally the opening of areas of capillary closure is noted, particularly at the macula, as revealed by fluorescein fundus photography (Archer *et al.*, 1970). Other, more general effects of photocoagulation are a decrease in the disten-

sion of the veins with a smoothing of their caliber and, as mentioned before, the production of a mild optic atrophy (Fig. 8-39).

Now, let us examine more closely the available statistical studies and my own results. Although we all known that the progression of the disease is often unequal in the two eyes, it is only by treating one eye in patients with early symmetrical diabetic retinopathy that the effect of photocoagulation can be established, since there are too many variables in the comparison of the eyes of one patient with the eyes of another, similarly affected patient (Irvine and Norton, 1971; Okun *et al.*, 1971; Hill, 1972; Freyler, 1974). As a rule, therefore, only series concerning patients in which one eye was treated and the other left as control, while the condition in both was of approximately the same type and degree, have been considered for review.

In my experience the effect of photocoagulation upon the waxy exudates and macular edema of the exudative type of background retinopathy has been less striking than in the reports in literature (Schott, 1964; Dobree, 1970*b*). While most workers express themselves in terms of a significant degree or complete disappearance of lesions, my experience is that although resorption of retinal edema and of lipoid deposits does occur frequently, this is by no means invariably so. Zweng *et al.* (1971) claim that the visual prognosis tends to be better in cases where only a localized leakage of fluid can be demonstrated angiographically than in those where there is diffuse leakage. Recently, Ticho and Patz (1973) have shown that the state of preoperative capillary perfusion as revealed by fluorescein fundus photography shows a close correlation with postoperative acuity results. Thus, good macular perfusion seems to be essential for the resolution of the edema fluid. In addition, cystoid collection of the dye at the posterior pole is generally a poor prognostic sign. Confirmation of this by other observers has made angiography an indispensable prognostic tool in every case of diabetic maculopathy.

In the hemorrhagic variety of simple diabetic retinopathy, an amelioration was seen in many cases, even if a number of them continued to deteriorate. This amelioration took the form of an attenuation of the distented veins with a reduction of beading, a decreased stagnation (even if the circulation time remained abnormal), a diminished retention of fluorescein by the vascular wall and a lessened incidence of bleeding episodes. In only three cases have I seen a proliferative retinopathy develop in an eye treated for preproliferative lesions. The rarity of this has also been under-

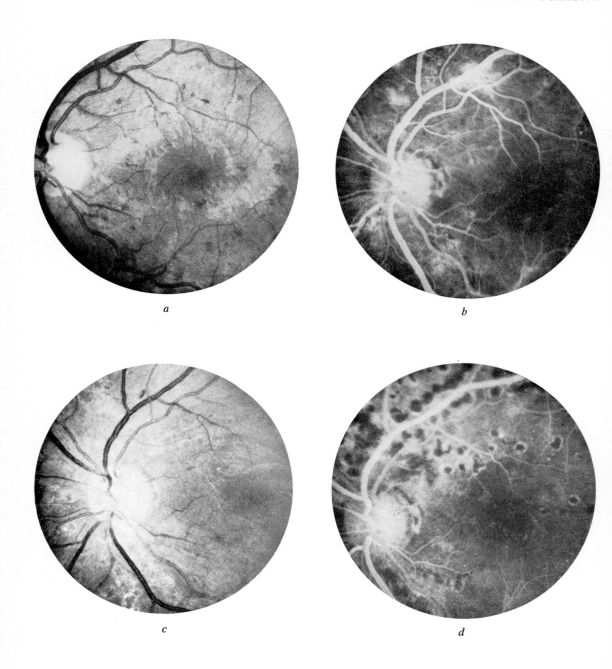

a

b

c

d

Fig. 8-39. — *a*) Left fundus of a 28-year-old man with diabetes of 18 years duration. Only a few scattered minute hemorrhages may be seen, plus a moderate, slightly irregular turgescence of the larger retinal veins and their main branches. Visual acuity: 5/5. *b*) In the late venous phase angiogram venous lesions become more apparent; the dye has left the vessels in several points and leaked into the overlying vitreous. *c*) Sixteen months after argon laser treatment there are only a few round hemorrhages left. The venous changes have regressed in part. Scarring is mild. The existing pallor of disc is indicative of descending optic atrophy. Visual acuity: 5/5. *d*) A late venous phase fluorescein angiogram shows complete atrophy of retinal capillaries at the photocoagulation marks. There no longer is any extravasation of dye.

scored by Meyer-Schwickerath and Schott (1968).

All in all, an analysis of the results obtained in 72 unilaterally photocoagulated patients of mine with nonproliferative symmetrical diabetic retinopathy, in whom the eye to be treated was chosen at random and who were kept under observation for no less than 24 months, reveals that the treated eyes fared better than their mates (Tables I and II).

The same may be said of those cases with a pro-

The information presented is in close agreement with the data in the studies cited above; it is at variance, however, with those of Irvine and Norton (1971) and of Borgmann *et al.* (1974), whose results have in the main been discouraging. The latter authors have shown that even if objective methods of evaluation are used in assessing progression or regression of the various features of diabetic retinopathy, one should always allow a

TABLE I. — MORPHOLOGICAL CHANGES AFTER UNILATERAL PHOTOCOAGULATION IN 72 CASES OF SYMMETRICAL BACKGROUND DIABETIC RETINOPATHY. FOLLOW-UP PERIOD 24 TO 121 MONTHS (AVERAGE 39 MONTHS) *.

	Treated eyes	Nontreated eyes
Improvement ..	47 (65.3 %)	2 (2.8 %)
No change ...	17 (23.6 %)	49 (68.0 %)
Impairment ...	8 (11.1 %)	21 (29.2 %)

* The results in each case were assessed by means of the Airlie House grading system.

TABLE II. — VISUAL RESULTS OF UNILATERAL PHOTOCOAGULATION IN 72 CASES OF SYMMETRICAL BACKGROUND DIABETIC RETINOPATHY. FOLLOW-UP PERIOD 24 TO 121 MONTHS (AVERAGE 39 MONTHS) *.

	Treated eyes	Nontreated eyes
Improvement .	3 (4.2 %)	0 (0.0 %)
No change ...	58 (80.5 %)	29 (40.2 %)
Impairment ...	11 (15.3 %)	43 (59.8 %)

* A difference of at least two lines on the Snellen chart was deemed necessary to classify an eye as improved or impaired.

liferative retinopathy. Both from a morphological and a visual standpoint, photocoagulation has proved to be profitable in the controlled studies of Okun (1968), Okun *et al.* (1971), Zetterstrom (1972), Dellaporta and Declercq (1973) and L'Esperance (1973). If we turn to the writer's material, which comprises 177 uniocularly treated patients divided into three categories, it can be said that the structural results were good in the case of the epiretinal and preretinal types of neovascularization, good, though less so, in the case of the epipapillary and prepapillary types of neovascularization, and rather uneven but still definitely encouraging in that of the papillovitreal and retinovitreal types (Tables III through VI).

wide margin for error. I have had no occasion to treat any of those cases of diabetic retinopathy with gross retinal ischemia which have been described by Bresnick *et al.* (1975), where photocoagulation — at least extensive photocoagulation — tends to exacerbate the vaso-obliterative process and usually results in a further visual decrement.

As to the effects of photocoagulation on vision in the proliferative form of the disease, the reader is referred to Fig. 8-40, where the varying mean acuities of both the treated eyes and the untreated fellow eyes are represented graphically (Urrets-Zavalía, 1974). It will be seen that, again, deterioration was less marked, and occurred more

TABLE III. — OVERALL MORPHOLOGICAL RESULTS OF UNILATERAL PHOTOCOAGULATION IN 177 CASES OF SYMMETRICAL PROLIFERATIVE DIABETIC RETINOPATHY. FOLLOW-UP PERIOD 12 TO 121 MONTHS (AVERAGE 23.3 MONTHS) *.

	Treated eyes	Nontreated eyes
Improvement .	87 (49.2 %)	2 (1.1 %)
No change ..	31 (17.5 %)	27 (15.3 %)
Progression ..	59 (33.3 %)	148 (83.6 %)
Stabilization **	118 (66.7 %)	29 (16.4 %)

* Whenever possible, the results were assessed by means of the Airlie House grading system.
** Improvement + no change.

TABLE IV. — MORPHOLOGICAL CHANGES AFTER UNILATERAL PHOTOCOAGULATION IN 31 CASES OF SYMMETRICAL PROLIFERATIVE DIABETIC RETINOPATHY: EPIRETINAL OR SURFACE NEOVASCULARIZATION ALONE. FOLLOW-UP PERIOD 12 TO 121 MONTHS (AVERAGE 35 MONTHS) *.

	Treated eyes	Nontreated eyes
Improvement ..	20 (64.5 %)	1 (3.2 %)
No change	3 (9.7 %)	1 (3.2 %)
Progression ...	8 (25.8 %)	29 (93.6 %)
Stabilization **	23 (74.2 %)	2 (6.4 %)

* Whenever possible, the results were assessed by means of the Airlie House grading system.
** Improvement + no change.

slowly in the treated eyes than in the untreated ones. In a review by Dobree and Taylor (1973) the data obtained in 174 eyes from 126 consecutive patients treated with xenon photocoagulation were compared with those in 59 control eyes from 42 patients. The authors considered solely the number

TABLE V. — MORPHOLOGICAL CHANGES AFTER UNI-LATERAL PHOTOCOAGULATION IN 56 CASES OF SYMME-TRICAL PROLIFERATIVE DIABETIC RETINOPATHY: EPIPA-PILLARY NEOVASCULARIZATION, ALONE OR COMBINED WITH EPIRETINAL NEOVASCULARIZATION. FOLLOW-UP PERIOD 12 TO 86 MONTHS (AVERAGE 27 MONTHS) *.

	Treated eyes	Nontreated eyes
Improvement ..	29 (51.8 %)	1 (1.8 %)
No change	8 (14.3 %)	8 (14.3 %)
Progression ...	19 (33.9 %)	47 (83.9 %)
Stabilization **	37 (66.1 %)	9 (16.1 %)

* Whenever possible, the results were assessed by means of the Airlie House grading system.
** Improvement + no change.

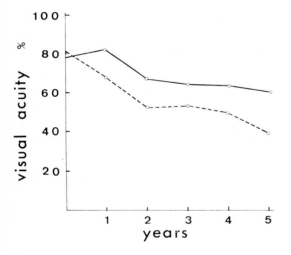

FIG. 8-40. — Changes in central vision undergone by 168 uniocularly treated patients with symmetrical proliferative diabetic retinopathy. Upper curve: treated eyes. Lower curve: control eyes.

of eyes retaining the same level of vision in each group at the end of one year, two years, and so on up to five years. It was seen that at all stages the treated eyes had a much better retention of vision than the controls, and that a high number retained their original acuity for over five years. Although

expressed in a different way, the results by Okun *et al.* (1971) are similar.

At the time that the above statistics were compiled I had been using the argon laser photocoagulator for only two years. Until then the results obtained in the treatment of the epipapillary, pa-

TABLE VI. — MORPHOLOGICAL CHANGES AFTER UNILATERAL PHOTOCOAGULATION IN 90 CASES OF SYMMETRICAL PROLIFERATIVE DIABETIC RETINOPATHY: PAPILLORETINAL AND/OR RETINOVITREAL NEOVASCULARIZATION. FOLLOW-UP PERIOD 12 TO 46 MONTHS (AVERAGE 17 MONTHS) *.

	Treated eyes	Nontreated eyes
Improvement ..	38 (42.2 %)	0 (0.0 %)
No change	20 (22.2 %)	18 (20.0 %)
Progression ..	32 (35.6 %)	72 (80.0 %)
Stabilization **	58 (64.4 %)	18 (20.0 %)

* Whenever possible, the results were assessed by means of the Airlie House grading system.
** Improvement + no change.

pillovitreal, and retinovitreal types of neovascular proliferation had been for the most part superior to the results obtained previously with the xenon-arc photocoagulator. Lacking an adequate perspective, as the observation period in the case of the patients treated with the argon laser was too short, I could not regard those results as proper statistical material and had to limit myself to mentioning the fact. From both the studies of Okun *et al.* (1971) and of Dobree and Taylor (1973) it appears that once the patient gets by the first two years after treatment, he tends to remain the same for at least five years as most failures occur rather early in the course of the follow-up period. Hence, it seemed that the gains for which the use of the argon laser had so far been responsible might be permanent and not ephemeral. Three more years of experience with the same instrument and a longer follow-up of those patients from the original 177 in Table III as returned for further examination served to cool somewhat my initial enthusiasm, and showed thet even after an uneventfull two post-treatment years, deterioration continued to occur, though at a slower pace (Table VII). The difference between the fate of the treated eyes and that of the untreated eyes remained no less striking, however.

Only after the returns of the long-term, multicenter cooperative trials that are under way in

TABLE VII. — OVERALL MORPHOLOGICAL RESULTS OF UNILATERAL PHOTOCOAGULATION IN 111 PATIENTS WITH SYMMETRICAL DIABETIC RETINOPATHY WHO RE-TURNED FOR FURTHER EXAMINATION DURING AN ADDITIONAL 36-MONTH PERIOD. ALL THESE CASES WERE PART OF THE ORIGINAL 177 CASES IN TABLE III. FOLLOW-UP PERIOD 48 TO 144 MONTHS (AVERAGE 66.2 MONTHS) *.

	Treated eyes	Nontreated eyes
Improvement ..	21 (18.9 %)	1 (0.9 %)
No change	27 (24.3 %)	8 (7.2 %)
Progression ...	63 (56.8 %)	102 (91.9 %)
Stabilization **	48 (43.2 %)	9 (8.1 %)

* Whenever possible, the results were assessed by means of the Airlie House grading system.
** Improvement + no change.

Great Britain and the United States are published, will a duly qualified answer be given to the question of whether photocoagulation can help prevent severe visual loss in diabetic retinopathy. Nevertheless it is possible to anticipate, in accordance with the rather universal results of those with even a modicum of experience, that the answer will be largely in the affirmative *.

In an effort to evaluate the relationship between the response to photocoagulation of proliferative retinopathy in the juvenile diabetic and the plasma growth hormone level, seven unilaterally treated patients in whom the results have been poor, six patients treated unilaterally with good results, and five healthy medical students who served as controls were studied during a 24-hour period with a precise radioimmunological technique (Ørskow *et al.*, 1968). Their ages ranged from 19 to 25 years (mean 22.4 years). The results obtained were as follows: In the first group the mean values were very high and the pattern was characterized by at least two steep peaks; in the second group the values were lower, though still abnormally elevated, and a base level could be recognized; in the controls, of course, the usual basal line with moderate peaks was found (Fig. 8-41). Thus patients with high and irregular plasma growth hormone levels have a poorer prognosis.

To appraise the role played by high blood pressure in the evolution of eyes suffering from the preproliferative (hemorrhagic) and proliferative forms that were treated with photocoagulation, a comparison was made of the values for the systolic pressure in 142 patients who reacted favorably with those in 207 patients who did not (Fig. 8-42). By displaying prominently the differences between the two groups, the curves indicate that high blood pressure exerts a pernicious influence on the course of diabetic retinopathy, even if it is not a factor in the pathogenesis of those changes that may be regarded as primary. Also, the difference in both curves suggests that a lowered blood pressure has a protective influence on the hemorrhagic progression of the disease.

The above figures concerning the level of growth hormone and blood pressure do not necessarily mean that photocoagulation should be withheld in favor of pituitary ablation or of purely medical treatment. They only mean that one must be cautious and know (*a*) that the prognosis varies in accordance with extraocular factors, (*b*) that the patient's cardiocirculatory conditions cannot be ignored, and (*c*) that in the case of a malignant retinopathy which does not respond favorably to

* An interim account of the Multicenter Controlled Photocoagulation Trial sponsored by the British Diabetic Association appeared while this book was in press (*Lancet* 2:1110, 1975). It reports the visual acuity results obtained in patients with diabetic maculopathy who were treated uniocularly with xenon-arc photocoagulation. Seventy-six patients were seen after one year, 44 after two years, and 25 after three years. The treated eyes retained significantly better visual acuity than the untreated ones. Eight treated vs. 18 untreated eyes became blind.

Another interim analysis of the cases in the same Multicenter Trial was prepared by H. Cheng (*Trans. ophthal. Soc. U.K.* 95:531, 1975); it also shows that treated eyes with maculopathy retain better visual acuity than untreated eyes. Furthermore, it shows that in cases with new vessels as the predominant feature, a significant difference in visual acuity between the treated and untreated eyes can be expected to occur if the trend observed so far continues to assert itself.

Quite lately, a preliminary report on the effect of both xenon-arc and argon laser photocoagulation was published in the United States by the Diabetic Retinopathy Study Research Group (*Amer. J. Ophthal.* 8:383, 1976). The results provide evidence that photocoagulation carried out in the form of either extensive scatter or a focal treatment of new vessels is of benefit in reducing, but not entirely eliminating, the risk of severe visual loss over a two-year period in eyes with proliferative retinopathy. The occurrence of visual acuity less than 5/200 for two consecutively completed four-month follow-up visits was thus reduced from 16.3 % in all untreated eyes to 6.4 % in all treated eyes. Although the information beyond two years of follow-up was limited, there was a continued reduction in the occurrence of severe visual loss in treated eyes as compared to untreated eyes. The same preliminary report showed that location of new vessels relative to the disc, severity of new vessels, and the presence of hemorrhage (vitreous or preretinal) all proved to be important prognostic factors.

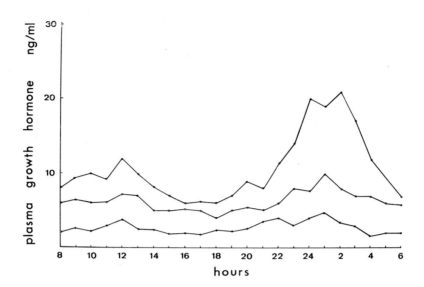

FIG. 8-41. — Mean diurnal patterns of plasma growth hormone. Upper curve: unilaterally photocoagulated symmetrical proliferative retinopathy in seven juvenile diabetics who reacted poorly or not at all. Middle curve: unilaterally photocoagulated symmetrical proliferative retinopathy in six juvenile diabetics in whom stabilization was achieved. Lower curve: five nondiabetic medical students used as controls.

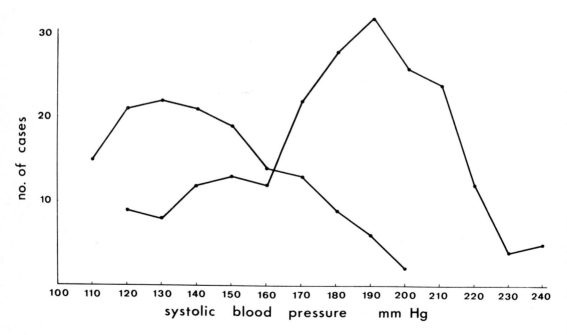

FIG. 8-42. — Systolic blood pressure curve in maturity-onset diabetics (age range 37 to 77 years, mean 59.7 years) suffering from severe preproliferative (hemorrhagic) or proliferative retinopathy. The line on the right side corresponds to 207 patients who did not respond well to light coagulation; the line on the left side to 142 patients in whom stabilization was achieved.

photocoagulation, a high level of plasma growth hormone may be an indication for hypophysectomy.

In conclusion, it would appear that if light coagulation has a definite place in the prevention or postponement of blindness in diabetic retinopathy, this place is dependent upon the clinical type of the disease, the stage at which light coagulation is applied, the plasma level of growth hormone, and the prevailing values of the blood pressure.

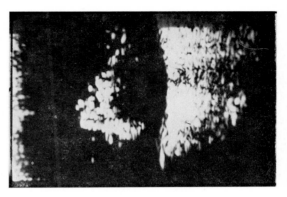

Fig. 8-44. — B-scan ultrasonogram of the eye shown in Fig. 8-43. The asteroid bodies appear as dense accoustic shadows in the vitreous cavity (80 dB).

DIFFICULTIES AND COMPLICATIONS OF PHOTOCOAGULATION

Among the difficulties that may hinder the performance of light coagulation in diabetic retinopathy one should mention:

1. Inadequate dilation of the pupil. This will interfere of course with the treatment of all but the most posteriorly located lesions.

2. Sclerosis or significant opacity of the lens.

3. Asteroid bodies in the vitreous gel. These seem to be more prevalent in diabetic than in nondiabetics, despite the assertion of Hatfield *et al.* (1962) to the contrary (Figs. 8-43 and 8-44).

The complications of xenon-arc photocoagulation are well known and have been dealt with by the author in a previous report (Urrets-Zavalía, 1968).

The complications that may appear after argon laser photocoagulation have been discussed in detail by Little and Zweng (1971), Little (1973*b*), and Zweng *et al.* (1974). Some of these, such as the corneal and lenticular burns due to an excessively high energy density, occur only exceptionally. Retinal hemorrhages are less rare and result (*a*) from the collision of a very narrow, high powered beam with a large vessel; (*b*) from the treatment of an epi- or juxtapapillary, densely packed cluster of new formed capillaries (Fig. 8-45); (*c*) from the obliteration of the efferent vessels from a *rete mirabile* without first occluding the afferent vessels (Fig. 8-48); or (*d*) from the accidental coagulation of an underlying retinal vessel beyond the point of focus upon an elevated, intravitreal vessel. Occasionally, a hemorrhage may be caused by the application of excessive coagulation intensity to an apparently avascular retinal spot. Zweng *et al.* (1974) found that the greatest number of complications seen among their diabetics consisted of hemorrhages occuring either at the time of treatment or up to one week later. In my experience, however, bleeding episodes related to photocoagulation have been seen only a few times and were almost always without gravity.

Fatigue or inattention on the part of the surgeon may cause a coagulation to go astray and hit the macula near the fovea.

Nerve fiber bundle defects are ordinarily associated with repeated photocoagulation about the optic disc. Thermal papillitis results form heavy photocoagulation directed at the nervehead itself,

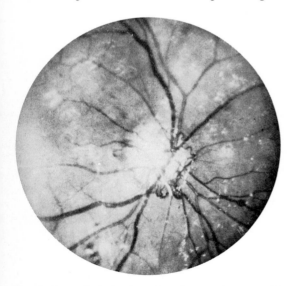

Fig. 8-43. — Left fundus of a 67-year-old man with diabetes of approximately 25 years duration. Early epi- and peripapillary neovascularization is present. There is marked asteroid hyalosis.

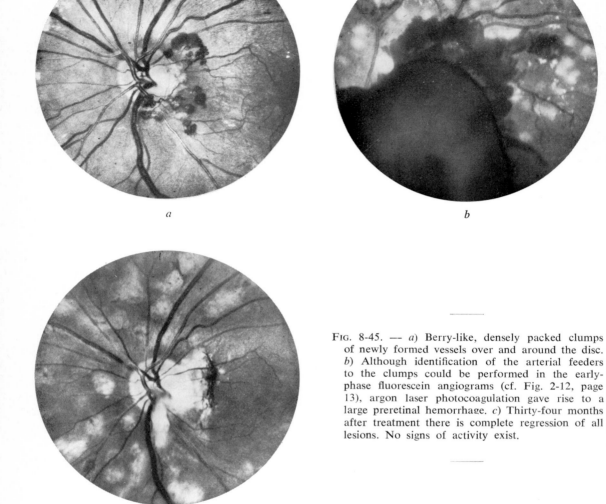

a

b

c

Fig. 8-45. — *a*) Berry-like, densely packed clumps of newly formed vessels over and around the disc. *b*) Although identification of the arterial feeders to the clumps could be performed in the early-phase fluorescein angiograms (cf. Fig. 2-12, page 13), argon laser photocoagulation gave rise to a large preretinal hemorrhage. *c*) Thirty-four months after treatment there is complete regression of all lesions. No signs of activity exist.

which becomes pale and swollen in the hours following photocoagulation. A marked improvement occurs within a few days, particularly if corticosteroids are given.

As already mentioned, the development of an epiretinal membrane over the macular region with subsequent contracture and a marked drop in visual acuity is not uncommon in elderly patients suffering from the exudative type of retinopathy. It can be avoided if only a limited amount of radiation is delivered to the posterior pole. When the slit-lamp discloses the presence of retinal edema or of microcystoid changes one knows that the fovea must be approached warily. The occurrence of a transient retinal detachment has been observed after heavy xenon or argon laser photocoagulation directed at the posterior pole. Although alarming for both the patient and surgeon, this *ablatio fugax*

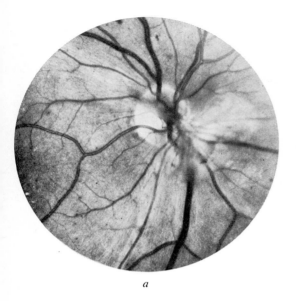

a

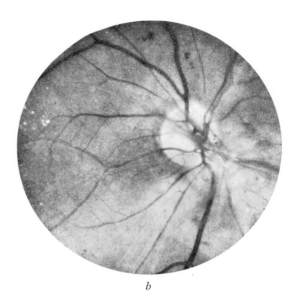

b

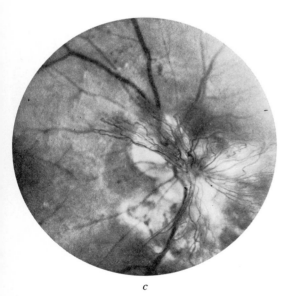

c

FIG. 8-46. — *a*) Right eye of a 72-year-old woman with diabetes of at least 30 years duration. Pre- and peripapillary neovascularization, immediately following xenon-arc photocoagulation. *b*) Eighteen months afterward there is complete elimination of all new vessels. *c*) After an additional two years there is extensive recurrence of the neovascularization which reaches into the vitreous at the level of, and beyond, the old photocoagulation scar.

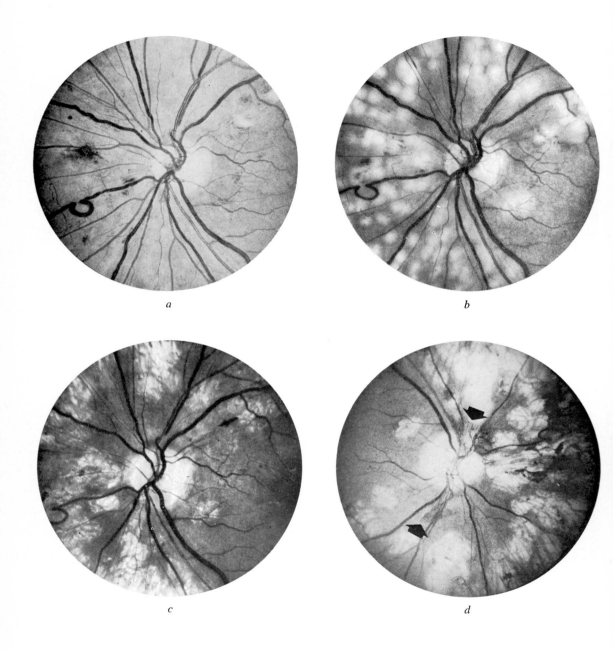

Fig. 8-47. — *a*) Left eye of a 27-year-old female, with diabetes of 24 years duration. Note engorgement of the veins with an omega-shaped loop at the 8 o'clock position, some wispy isolated epiretinal new vessels, scattered dot and blot hemorrhages, and a few cotton-wool spots. *b*) Same eye, 24 hours after completion of pan-retinal argon laser photocoagulation. *c*) Fifteen months later. Note the marked reduction in the caliber of the veins, obliteration of neovascularization and discrete pallor of the disc. *d*) One year afterward, an extensive though tenuous, tendril-like neovascularization has developed at the optic disc (arrows).

clears up spontaneously in a few days with restoration of the previous visual acuity (v. Barsewisch, 1971; Mautner, 1974). Less common but no less alarming is the development of a serous choroidal detachment which appears as the usual smooth-domed, single or multiple, bullous mound of choroid covered by closely adherent retina at the periphery of the fundus. Transillumination serves to differentiate it from a hemorrhagic detachment or a pigmented neoplasm. No treatment is required as all such detachments resolve spontaneously. Aphakic eyes are the most prone to this complication, which I have encountered only in the aged.

Less known but of considerable severity is the aggravation of a pre-existing rubeosis of the iris when the laser beam strikes it near the pupillary border due to insufficient mydriasis. Such an accident may remain unobserved until a sudden rise in pressure leads one to notice the neovascularized, atrophic patches in the mesodermal layers. On the other hand, it has been reported that elimination of new vessels on the retina exerts a favorable effect on rubeosis of the iris (Cleasby, 1968). This must be unusual for the remark is unique.

Rather than a complication, recurrent retinal neovascularization following repeated coagulation constitutes a failure (Fig. 8-46). Its ocurrence does not necessarily imply that the extent of the chorioretinal burns has been insufficient, for it may be observed in eyes where only the posterior pole was left untreated (Fig. 8-47). The fact that the stimulus for the formation of new vessels is still operative reveals that there are cases which cannot be managed with photocoagulation, even when this is applied early in the course of the disease; indeed, it looks sometimes as if with photocoagulation one merely succeeded in fertilizing the ground for neovascularization.

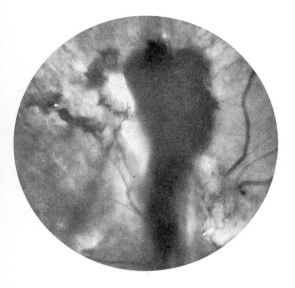

Fig. 8-48. — The same eye as shown in Fig. 8-36 (page 81) after treatment of the large neovascular fan located superiorly. Argon laser photocoagulation of the feeder vessels found in the angiogram was obviously ineffective in arresting the blood flow into the fan, which then bled profusely as it was approached with the 500 μ size spot.

CHAPTER 9

SCLERAL AND VITREOUS SURGERY IN THE MANAGEMENT OF PROLIFERATIVE DIABETIC RETINOPATHY AND ITS COMPLICATIONS

Let us consider now those surgical procedures that can be of help in the case of some of the more severe retinal complications of proliferative diabetic retinopathy: scleral diathermy coagulation; the scleroplastic operations, which are being used for traction retinal detachment, either nonrhegmatogenous or rhegmatogenous; the vitrectomy procedures through both the posterior and the anterior routes; and, more as an adjunct to vitrectomy than as an independent procedure, endodiathermy.

SCLERAL DIATHERMY COAGULATION IN THE TREATMENT OF DIABETIC RETINOPATHY

With the hope of duplicating some conditions which result in chorioretinal atrophy, where the occurrence of diabetic retinopathy is rare, Amalric (1960-1967) used transscleral diathermy in the form a large band of isolated coagulations extending from the equator backward over two or three quadrants. An amelioration was reported in a limited number of cases of nonproliferative retinopathy of the exudative type; in others, the prompt resolution of massive intravitreal hemorrhage could be seen, a fact which had previously been noted by Verhoeff (1947) in a single instance of Eale's disease, and by Franceschetti (1955) in eight.

More recently, Wessing and Böckenhoff (1971) reported on the results of intrascleral diathermy in proliferative retinopathy. In approximately half of their cases the procedure succeeded in curbing the intravitreal proliferation of vessels; no data concerning the lenght of the observation period are given. In a vast majority (21 out of 23) of those cases with a massive hemorrhage of less than two months' duration, it brought about a rapid resorption of the blood in the vitreous body.

The technique is as follows: An incision is made through the conjunctiva and Tenon's capsule over the temporal semicircumference. Once the sclera is bared of all adhesions, the anterior limit of the area to be treated is outlined at the equator with a knife or other suitable instrument, and the outer two-thirds of the scleral thickness are separated from the inner third over a crescent 4 mm in width. The entire thinned area is coagulated lightly with diathermy from a ball electrode, the lamellar flap is replaced, and the incision reunited with a number of separate sutures or with a biological adhesive such as a butyl-cyano-acrylate. Finally, the conjunctiva and Tenon's are closed with a running suture.

However, in my experience, which comprises 14 eyes with proliferative retinopathy and a clear vitreous that were operated upon from 1961 through 1969, there has not been a single case in which quiescence resulted from the application of transscleral or intrascleral diathermy. In a randomized series of 21 additional eyes with a copious vitreous hemorrhage of no more than three month's duration, the 11 eyes that were treated had no better fortune than the ten eyes that were left untreated. Thus it would seem that the favorable results obtained by Wessing and Böckenhoff in the cases of seemingly arrested neovascularization may simply have represented an insufficient follow-up; the resolution of intraocular hemorrhages may merely demonstrate the propensity of most fresh collections of blood to clear up in a relatively short time.

SECTION
OF THE POSTERIOR SCLERAL RING
AND CANAL

Working on the unproven assumption that diabetic retinopathy is primarily due to venous stasis, and that it is at the posterior scleral ring and canal that the blood flow in the vena centralis encounters the most difficulty, Vasco Posada (1970, 1972) has devised a surgical technique wherein the posterior segment of the globe is approached by the anterior nasal route, and an incision made through the posterior scleral ring and canal, and through the dura of the optic nerve. Improved drainage should result in rapid improvement of the retinal condition, even in its late proliferation stages. Cessation of bleeding and regression of the neovascular systems would be among the most striking changes.

Although I have had no personal experience with this procedure, I believe that it should be given the benefit of a controlled trial.

SURGERY FOR RETINAL DETACHMENT
IN COMPLICATED
DIABETIC RETINOPATHY

Perhaps the most fearsome sequela of fibrotic proliferation with late shrinkage is the development of retinal detachment (Pannarale, 1969; Okun and Fung, 1969; McMeel, 1971; Olivella, 1972; Boniuk *et al.*, 1972; Tasman, 1972). As traction develops the retina separates from the pigment epithelium behind the equator and becomes tented up. Characteristically, the pull into the vitreous cavity is perpendicular to the retinal surface although it may be tangential. The elevated retina is rigid and the progression of the detachment is slow. The effect on vision depends on whether or not the macula is involved. As soon as a break occurs, usually as a result of centripetal traction, the detachment extends rapidly and acquires the features of the rhegmatogenous type. As a rule, the retinal breaks appear in the vicinity of the disc and are oval in shape (Fig. 9-1); there may be some kinking of the adjacent vessels, revealing that there is either a vitreous tug or a drag by an epiretinal membrane.

As long as the detachment remains localized and

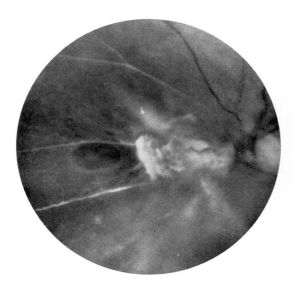

FIG. 9-1. — Typical retinal hole in a subtotal diabetic traction detachment. Note the oval contour, posterior location, and close proximity to a dense epiretinal membrane and to several obliterated vessels.

the macula is not threatened, surgery may be delayed and the patient examined every few months. Extension to the macula with a drop in visual acuity makes immediate surgery imperative.

In the nonrhegmatognous variety of detachment the consensus is that a lamellar scleral resection over at least two quadrants or an encircling buckling procedure in the region of the equator with a silicone band or rod should be performed, to release some of the traction on the detached retina and let it settle back into place (Figs. 9-2 and 9-3). As pointed out by Okun *et al.* (1971) drainage of subretinal fluid is not only dangerous, in that sudden hypotony may predispose to an intraocular hemorrhage, but unnecessary, for the retina will flatten by itself if the intraocular pressure is brought to a level of approximately 30-35 mm Hg. If a retinal hole exists, an encirclement should also be effected in order to relieve traction by indenting the sclera, and an associated segmental implant — preferably an episcleral silicone sponge — affixed by one or two mattress sutures over the existing break. At the end of the procedure if the subretinal fluid is drained, or as soon as the retina settles upon the posteriorly located buckle, the margins of the hole must be photocoagulated (Fig. 9-4). An added benefit of this operation lies in the fact that, as the intravitreal

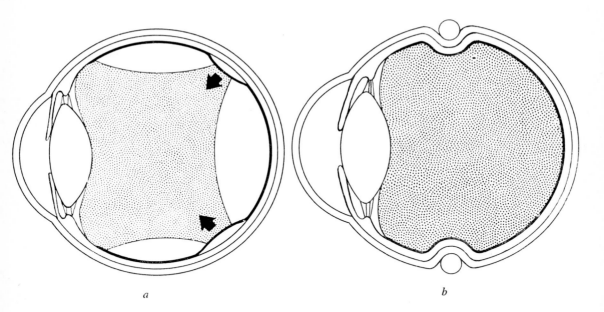

a   b

FIG. 9-2. — *a*) Schematic representation of nonrhegmatogenous retinal detachment due to traction exerted by shrinking vitreous. *b*) Permanent encirclement of globe with nonresorbable material relieves traction and leads to reattachment of retina.

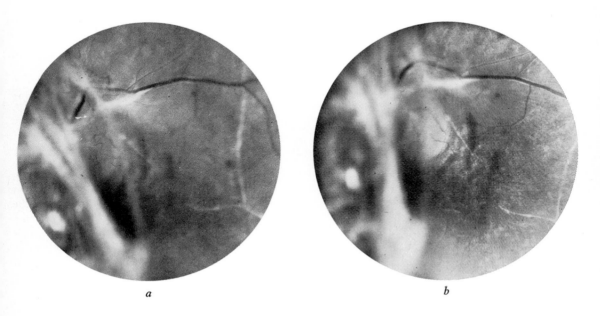

a   b

FIG. 9-3. — *a*) A flat, rigid retinal detachment of the nonrhegmatogenous variety due to tangential traction exerted by a dense connective membrane overlying the disc. Note sheathing of vein and linear proliferation of glia. Visual acuity: hand movements at 1 m. *b*) Total reattachment of the retina following encirclement with a silicone band. Postoperative corrected visual acuity: 5/40.

new vessels collapse, bleeding ceases and the vitreous clears up (Wetzig, 1972). Moreover, it should be noted that the procedure is virtually without risks and that its execution offers no special difficulties.

Some two-thirds of the reported cases have shown a definite improvement, and this regardless of whether any retinal breaks were present. Though far from being uniformly bad, my own experience has been much less encouraging. Out of 13 cases of nonrhegmatogenous and six of rhegmatogenous detachments treated by cerclage

VITRECTOMY
THROUGH THE POSTERIOR ROUTE

The instrumentation for the surgical removal of the vitreous through the *pars plana ciliaris* and the technique in use have largely been developed by Machemer and his group (1971-1974a). Working independently, Klöti (1973, 1974) has devised an instrument which operates on a different principle, as have other authors in the

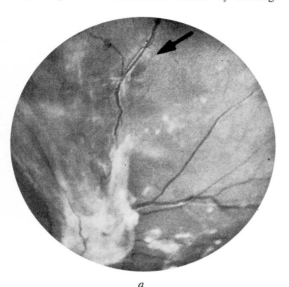

a

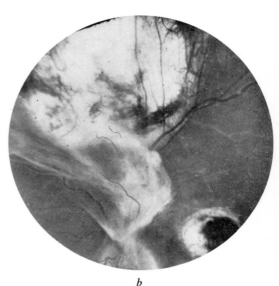

b

FIG. 9-4. — *a*) Flat traction retinal detachment due to an epipapillary membrane. Note the oval break lying alongside the radial vessel at 12 o'clock (arrow). *b*) The retina is in place, one year after encirclement, cryocoagulation, and episcleral plombage with a silicone sponge over the hole. The preretinal membrane is now lax and floats in the posterior vitreous cavity.

and (when necessary) a segmental implant, only four were cured after one year. In three the disease took an immediate turn for the worse, which consisted of an extension of the pre-existing neovascularization followed by repeated bleeding into the vitreous. In the remaining 12, the disease process seemed to proceed undisturbed, after showing sometimes a temporary reprieve. Accordingly, I have now all but abandoned the cerclages in favor of vitrectomy for the traction type of detachment, and use them sparingly in the rhegmatogenous type, where scleral buckling, either segmental of encircling, may represent the last important step in the performance of a pars plana vitrectomy.

course of the last couple of years (Douvas, 1973, 1975; Peyman *et al.*, 1973). The writer has had considerable first-hand experience with both the *vitreous-infusion-suction-cutter* (VISC) of Machemer and the *vitreous stripper* of Klöti. As regards the indications and results, that experience merely confirms the observations of Machemer (1973b) relating to this first 53 cases of complicated diabetic retinopathy.

The possible applications of subtotal vitrectomy in the treatment of diabetic retinopathy are manifold. It may be used to eliminate the blood in the vitreous cavity, after a waiting period of no less than six months following a profuse intraocular hemorrhage. It is seldom needed in the case of a first or even a second bleeding episode, where the extravasation is often inconsiderable and there is a tendency toward spontaneous resorption. More frequently, massive hemorrhages occur late in the course of the disease; they do not belong exclusively to the proliferative form and may be observed in eyes with no neovascularization whatsoever but with badly damaged veins and a number of large microaneurysms. It is in the latter type of case, in which there are no fibrovascular masses in the vitreous but only dense, more or less closely packed intravitreal fibrinous

so that fundus details are visible. The attack must be directed at the outer surface of the detached vitreous (Fig. 9-8). Although the retina may reattach spontaneously once the traction to which it was subjected disappears, an equatorial encirclage should be performed after the vitrectomy itself, and a segmental implant anchored at the site of any recognizable break.

Finally, vitrectomy may be used to nibble at the gross fibrovascular stalks that originate at the disc and advance freely into the vitreous. These constitute not only a visual obstruction but, until

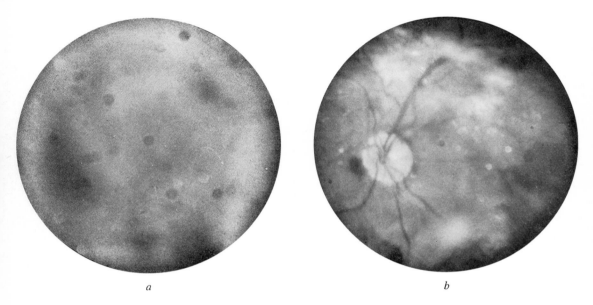

a   *b*

FIG. 9-5. — *a*) Right eye of a 54-year-old man with diabetes of 15 years duration. Because of recurrent vitreous hemorrhages only perception of light remains. The red fundus reflex can scarcely be seen. *b*) Seven months after vitrectomy through the pars plana with removal of proliferative membranes, only a slight vitreous haze persists. Visual acuity: 5/30.

clots, or blood pools located between the retina and vitreous, that the best results are obtained (Fig. 9-5). Traction by the vitreous on the new vessels arising from either the retina or the nervehead represents the most important single factor in the production of recurring intravitreal hemorrhages (Figs. 9-6 and 9-7). Thus, it is not surprising that once the pulling force has been removed by vitrectomy the abnormal vessels contract, shrivel and seem to lose some of their propensity to bleed.

As a means of relieving traction on the retina, vitrectomy finds an important indication in the management of secondary retinal detachment, particularly when the vitreous is still relatively clear,

the very last stages, a potential source of vitreous hemorrhage. The peeling off of an epiretinal membrane is more difficult; in experienced hands it may be brought to a successful conclusion by lifting up one edge of the membrane with an auxiliary instrument (Figs. 9-9 and 9-10). Yet it must be noted that neither the arciform bands that extend from the optic nervehead over the retinal surface nor the massive epiretinal organization that occurs in retinal detachment can always be approached in this way, for the arciform bands are largely subretinal, and the fibrous tissue that develops over the retina in the case of long-standing, funnel-shaped detachments or as a complication of retinal surgery is intimately connected with the retina and may actually have become part of it.

Before a patient may be accepted as a candidate for vitrectomy, evaluation of the remaining retinal function is crucial. Whenever possible, preoperative examination should include binocular indirect ophthalmoscopy, direct ophthalmoscopy, and slit-lamp biomicroscopy with the Goldmann three-mirror contact lens. In cases of lens or vitreous opacification, good light perception and projection are a good omen, as is also a positive red-green discrimination. Being unable to recognize entoptic phenomena myself, I have been unable to use them as a test of functioning retina; according to Machemer (1973*b*) they are useful, however, unless the opacification of the media is too dense. Macular function may be explored by means of the Maddox rod or through the simultaneous presentation of two lights, 10 to 30 cm apart, held at 1 m from the patient; here again, the ability to tell whether the light source appears as a vertical or horizontal line, or to discriminate between the two points will be abolished if the opacity of the lens or vitreous is very dense. With all its limitations, ultrasonography — especially B-

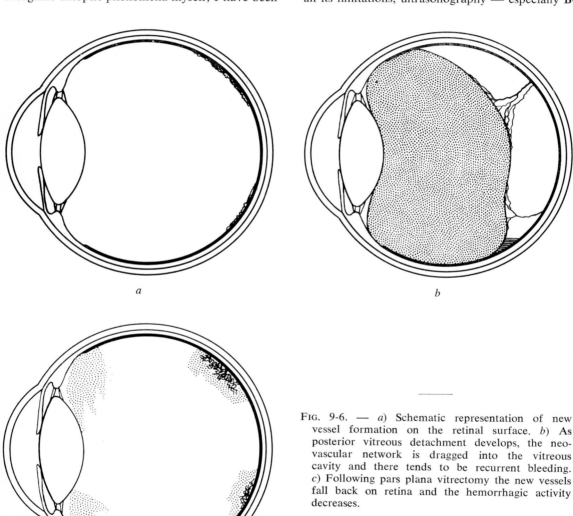

FIG. 9-6. — *a*) Schematic representation of new vessel formation on the retinal surface. *b*) As posterior vitreous detachment develops, the neovascular network is dragged into the vitreous cavity and there tends to be recurrent bleeding. *c*) Following pars plana vitrectomy the new vessels fall back on retina and the hemorrhagic activity decreases.

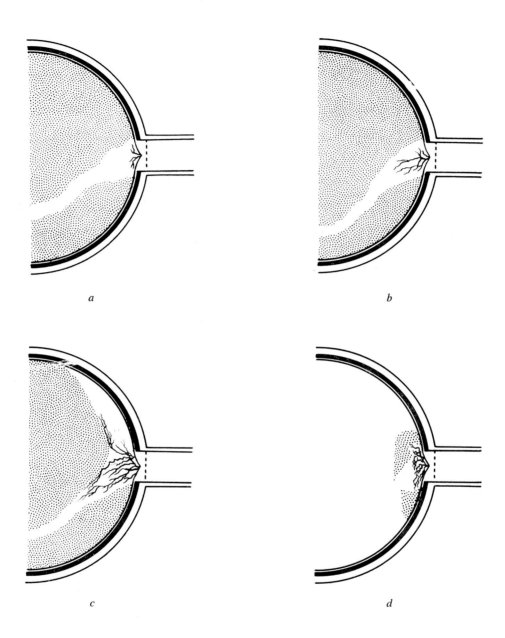

FIG. 9-7. — *a*) Schematic representation of early epipapillary neovascularization. *b*) Active growth of new formed vessels into the primary vitreous, which is fluid and not bound posteriorly by a limiting membrane. *c*) As neovascularization advances further anteriorly it becomes adherent to the plicata and the posterior limiting membrane, and is pulled forward as the vitreous becomes detached. This in turn causes repeated bleeding. *d*) After vitrectomy all traction ceases, the new vessels tend to shrivel and the hemorrhagic activity stops.

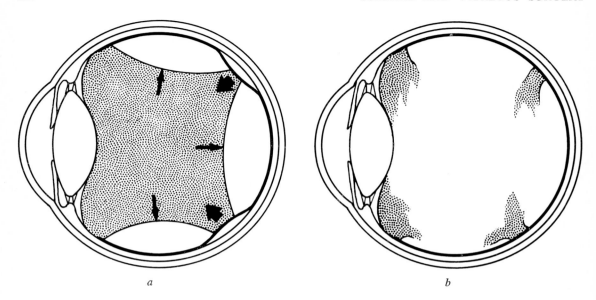

a   *b*

FIG. 9-8. — *a*) Schematic representation of both tangential and axial pull on the retina by rigid, retracted vitreous. *b*) After subtotal vitrectomy via the pars plana all traction on the retina has disappeared. Note that the vitreous base has been left undisturbed. (See text.)

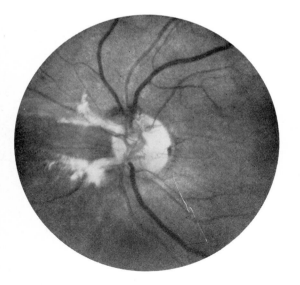

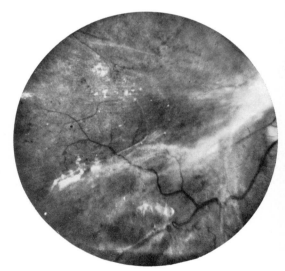

FIG. 9-9. — Left fundus of a 37-year-old woman one year after posterior vitrectomy for massive vitreous bleeding due to fibrovascular proliferations arising from the optic disc. Only a moderate vitreous haze, some epiretinal fibrous remnants and one juxtapapillary small hemorrhage remain. The preoperative vision was reduced to light perception with good projection; present vision is 5/15.

FIG. 9-10. — Right fundus of a 68-year-old woman 18 months after conventional cataract extraction followed by pars plana vitrectomy. Only some tenuous fibrous remnants were left over the papillomacular and macular regions. The preoperative vision was light perception with poor projection; corrected postoperative vision was 5/50 when last seen.

scan — is most helpful, particularly when the other tests fail to give the information required. It should be carried out by the surgeon himself in practically all cases (Jack *et al.*, 1974). The indications of bright-flash electroretinography have been discussed in p. 40.

Those interested in a detailed description of the surgical procedure are referred to the reports by Machemer and his coworkers and by Klöti cited above. In broad outline the technique is as follows.

A Remedi lid retractor or other adequate instrument is inserted, and the sclera is bared on the temporal side by an incision made through the conjunctiva and Tenon's capsule. Blunt dissection is used to expose the insertion of the lateral rectus and a silk traction suture is passed under that muscle. A superficial sclerotomy, parallel to and 5 mm distant from the limbus, is then performed on the temporal side, above or below the horizontal meridian, and a mattress suture using 5-0 white supramid placed through the edges of the incision.

Before the sclera is perforated, the corneal epithelium should be removed, as it would become cloudy during the operation and hinder visibility in the vitreous cavity. To this end, a few drops of absolute alcohol are instilled on the cornea; after only one minute the entire epithelium becomes loose and can be swept away with a cotton swab.

A modified plano-concave Goldmann contact lens is then affixed to the globe by means of three direct sutures. Holding the contact lens by the tube serving to inject saline between lens and cornea the surgeon may turn the eye in any desired position.

A special beveled knife is used to cut the remaining scleral layers and to prepare a track into the vitreous, so that the tip of the vitrectomy instrument does not tend to push the vitreous base and produce a pars plana detachment. A short pilot tube is then inserted into the eye and the mattress suture pulled tightly around the tube and temporarily tied. The vitrectomy instrument is introduced through the pilot tube and the removal of vitreous started in the axial region (Fig. 9-11). The operation is done under observation through the microscope at a power of 10 to 25. Illumination is provided by either a coaxial beam, a motorized slit-lamp or a fiberoptic sleeve. Ringer's solution is generally used to replace the removed vitreous and maintain intraocular volume. As a rule, suction is carried out by hand with a 30 ml syringe.

When all the desired vitreous, pooled blood, vitreous strands, and preretinal membranes have been removed the instrument is withdrawn and replaced by an infusion tube. This and the pilot tube are then retracted while the assistant pulls firmly on the two ends of the preplaced suture, which is subsequently tied and cut short. The

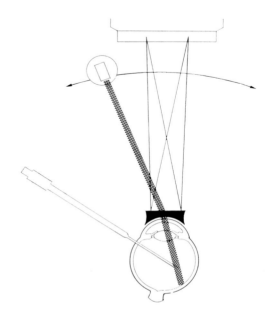

FIG. 9-11. — Schematic representation of the observation and external illumination systems used in pars plana vitrectomy. A plano-concave or wide-angle biconcave contact lens is in place. (After MACHEMER, 1973 *b*.)

stitches serving to attach the contact lens are cut and the conjunctival wound closed with a running silk suture.

General anesthesia (with halothane as the agent of choice) may be used in most cases. In some, however, with threatening renal failure, decompensated heart disease or other late complication of diabetes mellitus, neuroleptanalgesia is to be preferred. Used with regional anesthesia, neuroleptanalgesia is achieved through the intravenous or intramuscular injection of droperidol, a neuroleptic (tranquilizer) with antiemetic properties, and fentanyl, a potent narcotic analgesic. It will ensure the safe, smooth course of the procedure, which may last several hours, and it causes very few adverse reactions.

Vitrectomy is not without complications (Machemer and Norton, 1972*a* and *b*). Among those encountered at operation, the following may be recalled:

1. Damage to the lens capsule by the tip of the instrument, which should always be oriented toward the center of the vitreous cavity.

2. Avulsion of the retina at the ora serrata by the vitreous base. To avoid this, tunnelization of the vitreous with a large sclerotomy knife is imperative. Vitrectomy should never be pushed too near the vitreous base, where the vitreous is sticky and will adhere to the tip without being cut, thereby exercising traction on the pars plana and retina.

3. Production of retinal holes when working on a posteriorly located membrane, or a detached retina.

4. Persistent intravitreal bleeding, which cannot always be stopped permanently by elevating the infusion bottle in an effort to raise intraocular pressure above the systolic level. If necessary, intraocular, underwater diathermy must be used to coagulate the offending vessel.

5. Incarceration of organized vitreous or fibrous tissue into the suction hole of the tip. This immobilizes the cutting mechanism of the instrument. To free the tip, the assistant working the aspiration syringe should reverse aspiration while the surgeon slowly rotates the instrument along its long axis. If this fails, a fine Ziegler knife must be introduced through the pars plana into the vitreous cavity, at right angles to the instrument, and the adherent tissue cut off or teased with the blade from the tip. It may happen that after being disengaged the tip refuses to function, in which case it has to be withdrawn from the eye, dismantled and cleaned before being reintroduced.

6. The discovery of an unsuspected retinal detachment, whether rhegmatogenous or nonrheg-matogenous, particularly when the vitreous is still turbid, has a heavy demoralizing effect and calls for extreme caution if it is decided to go ahead with the operation. The ever present danger in such cases lies of course in the ease with which the free-floating retina can be aspirated into the tip and cut (Fig. 9-12). Repair of a preexisting retinal detachment after vitrectomy has been completed is not often successful even in experienced hands.

The main postoperative complications are as follows:

1. The presence of residual floaters is common and should be disregarded. Recurrent hemorrhage

into the vitreous may be copious and occurs not uncommonly, since the disease itself is not cured (Fig. 9-13). As a rule, resorption occurs more rapidly after vitrectomy than in the intact eye,

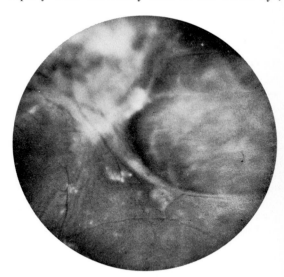

FIG. 9-12. — A large retinal break (upper right quadrant of figure) created through overenergetic suction due to inexperience, in an eye suffering from advanced proliferative diabetic retinopathy.

especially if the lens has been removed. This is due in part to the absence of any collagen or hyaluronic acid derivatives, and partly to the fact that after lensectomy blood and its breakdown products may escape though the anterior outflow channels.

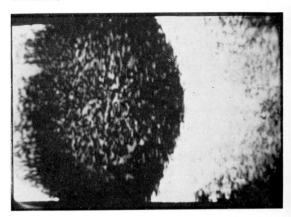

FIG. 9-13. — B-scan ultrasonogram of an eye with recurrent hemorrhage after vitrectomy. Note the uniform distribution of multiple small clots.

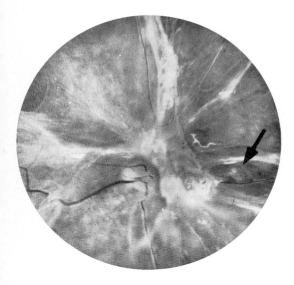

FIG. 9-14. — Right eye of a 65-year-old patient one year after vitrectomy for dense vitreous opacity in advanced proliferative retinopathy. Incomplete removal of the prepapillary avasculaı membrane was followed by shrinkage and formation of a retinal hole (arrows).

2. Residual fibrous tissue on the retinal surface may contract belatedly and lead to the formation of retinal holes near the disc, or to traction detachment involving the macula (Fig. 9-14). In some cases where the retinal surface seemed absolutely clear at the end of the procedure and remained so for some time postoperatively, I have seen one or more round or oval holes develop in an entirely flat retina (Fig. 9-15). Located for the most part at the posterior pole, these can readily be sealed with photocoagulation.

3. The late appearance of a rhegmatogenous retinal detachment after vitrectomy carries a bad prognosis, unless the peripheral vitreous happens to have cleared up considerably, which is unusual, and the break responsible for the detachment can be identified with reasonable certainty.

4. Cataract formation in a previously intact lens or the progression of old cataractous changes is a frequent although by no means invariably finding after vitrectomy for diabetic retinopathy. Removal of an opaque lens in the patient already submitted to a vitrectomy should be done by cryoextraction. Enzymatic zonulolysis is to be avoided, for the lens would sink from sight into

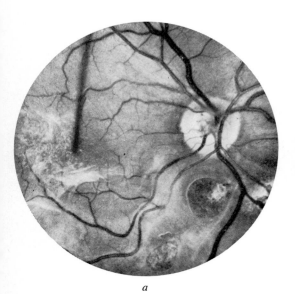

a

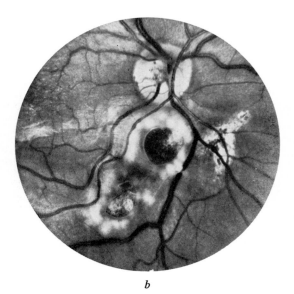

b

FIG. 9-15. — *a*) The right fundus of a 22-year-old patient with advanced proliferative retinopathy and a traction retinal detachment, four months after vitrectomy. The retinal surface is clear except for a thin epiretinal membrane over the macular area. There was late development of two round holes near disc. *b*) The same eye following argon laser photocoagulation. Note a small operative scar on the right of the upper hole.

the fluid which fills the vitreous compartment and become lost as soon as it is freed from its normal attachments.

5. Glaucoma, either hemolytic or open-angle, may complicate an otherwise uneventful postoperative course. The former is due to blockage of the trabecular meskwork by red cells and their debris. Diagnosis can readily be made by gonioscopy, which shows a reddish pigmentation of the trabecular meshwork. As the blood remnants desintegrate or are washed out of the eye, the intraocular pressure decreases spontaneously until it falls within normal limits. While it lasts, however, this form of glaucoma is easily controlled with acetazolamide and the instillation of epinephrine drops. The latter, non-hemolytic form of glaucoma occurs more rarely and responds less well to medical therapy; its pathogenesis is not clear.

The results vary with the severity of the underlying pathology. Cases of simple vitreous hemorrhage without proliferative retinopathy are very easy to treat and usually show spectacular improvement. When the vitreous contains not only scattered clots but also a hematogenous, avascular membrane in its posterior part, the prognosis is usually quite good. These membranes are yellow-ocher in color and go from one side of the eye

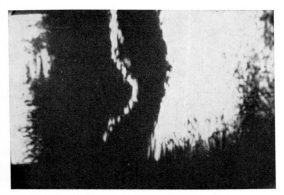

FIG. 9-16. — B-scan ultrasonogram of an eye with a simple vitreous hemorrhage due to maturity-onset, nonproliferative diabetic retinopathy. Note the typical, frontally oriented yellow-ocher membrane.

to the other; they tremble with the movements of the eye and never resorb spontaneously (Fig. 9-16). In patients with a hemorrhagic vitreous and retinitis proliferans but without retinal detachment the operation is more difficult to perform;

the success rate however remains high, at or about 70 %. When there is a retinal detachment in addition to vitreous opacity and intravitreal proliferans, the prognosis is extremely poor. My own experience with the resection of cloudy vitreous in the presence of retinal detachment has shown the results to vary with the nature of the latter. In traction detachment, where the retina is rather tense and its elevation from the pigment epithelium discrete, the difficulties encountered have not been too considerable. In rhegmatogenous detachment, mechanical separation of the opaque vitreous and fibrous tissue from the floating retina may be an all but impossible task. Also poor, although less so, is the prognosis in retinitis proliferans with secondary retinal detachment and a clear vitreous, where the initial results, often quite good, may be nullified after a while by the deterioration produced by a progression of the disease.

But if removal of old blood in the vitreous, the cutting of strands, and the removal of fibrovascular membranes are valuable, vitrectomy does more than that. As Machemer and Norton (1972b) have pointed out, by removing the vitreous the surface on which vessels can grow and the agent which pulls on them are eliminated. Future neovascular proliferation must spread along the retinal surface, where it will be free from traction and most vulnerable to photocoagulation.

Not every case of proliferative diabetic retinopathy with vitreous invasion and/or persistent turbidity should be summitted to vitrectomy. Contraindications are:

1. The absence of light perception.

2. A negative bright-flash ERG in the presence of an echographically attached retina.

3. The presence of extensive rubeosis, even if the intraocular pressure is normal.

4. The presence of a traction circumpapillary retinal detachment or of an extensive retinal detachment of the morning-glory type, where the disc is seen at the end of a tunnel formed by the agglutination of convergent retinal folds.

5. The presence of a florid proliferation at the posterior pole with numerous large vessels on the advancing sheets.

It is the feeling of many that in the event of a very active, densely vascularized proliferative retinopathy with a definite tendency to repeated bleeding, vitrectomy should be postponed one or even several years until the active stage of the disease burns itself out. After spontaneous occlusion af many of the new vessels has occurred the operation will have more chance of success. The argument is not entirely convincing, however, for when the disease is left to its own devices it may end by damaging the eye beyond all possibilities of repair (Fig. 9-17).

removal through the dilated and surgically enlarged pupil, attempts have been made to use the procedure in patients with severe and persistent vitreous hemorrhage due to diabetic retinopathy (Scott,

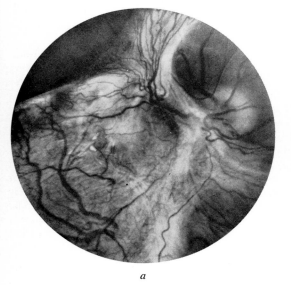

a

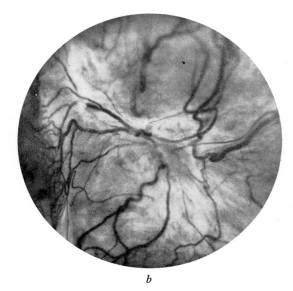

b

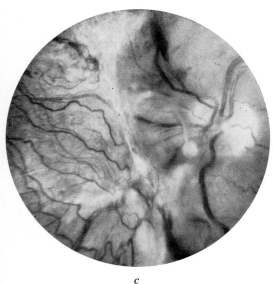

c

FIG. 9-17. — Some inoperable eyes. *a*) Right fundus of a 39-year-old man with diabetes of 17 years duration. The existing fibrovascular changes are too severe to be treated by either photocoagulation, vitrectomy, or pituitary ablation. *b*) Right fundus of a 56-year-old man with diabetes of 32 years duration. Due to massive proliferative retinopathy the normal landmarks are no longer recognizable. *c*) Left fundus of a 70-year-old man with diabetes of 18 years duration. A dense preretinal fibrovascular membrane covers the nasal retina. Visual acuity was still 5/20, as the macula showed a slight edema but was otherwise unaltered.

VITRECTOMY
THROUGH THE ANTERIOR ROUTE

Ever since Kasner *et al.* (1968) succeeded in treating amyloidosis of the vitreous in two patients through lens extraction followed by partial vitreous

1969, 1972, 1973; Shafer, 1972; van Heusen, 1972).

The operation requires that an operating microscope with coaxial illumination be used, and that a Flieringa ring of suitable size be affixed to the globe. Access to the anterior chamber is gained through a limbal section of about 270-300° or through an 8 mm trephine hole, the reclined cornea or excised corneal disc being placed in some sort of a moist chamber. The lens is removed using alpha-chymotrypsin and a cryoprobe, and the vitreous is excised layer by layer up to and including all thickened membranes and traction bands, and as much fibrovascular tissue as may be approached without endangering the retina.

A few dozen cases have been operated upon by several authors with varying degrees of success. To my mind, the so-called open-sky or transpupillary vitrectomy cannot compare with closed vitrectomy. The opening through which all maneuvers have to be carried out is narrow and the visibility poor. The instruments used through the posterior route are superior in their cutting ability to those which can be inserted through the pupil deep into the vitreous chamber. The stable pressure relationships which the new vitrectomy instruments help maintain, and the fact that they provide constant suction and infusion are also important, as is the ease with which a second instrument — needle for lavage or hook to lift up those epiretinal membranes that are to be removed — may be introduced into the eye and moved about under good visual control.

ENDODIATHERMY

Developed by Dellaporta (1951) as a means of sealing posteriorly located retinal holes or of coagulating neovascular fronds from the inside under ophthalmoscopic control, transvitreal diathermy has been revived by Shea (1972) with the same ends in view. Shea reported four cases of diabetic retinopathy which had proved resistant to argon laser photocoagulation and were subsequently treated with a stainless steel, teflon-insulated needle introduced through the pars plana. In three, the procedure was successful insofar as there was no vascular regrowth or recurrent hemorrhage during the follow-up period.

More recently, Klöti (1974) perfected a diathermy electrode and handle supplied with infusion and suction which can be introduced into the eye through the opening serving to insert the vitreous stripper. By keeping the vitreous chamber clear with continuous lavage, this permits an easier identification and closure of any persistently bleeding vessel during vitrectomy. In this case, of course, visual guidance of the instrument's tip and shaft is provided by the surgical microscope. For the electrode to be fully effective when entirely submerged, the frequency of the current should be of only 0.5-1.5 MHz. Because of their tendency to stray beyond all insulation, currents of a higher frequency such as are used in most diathermy units for retinal detachment are subject to great dispersion as soon as the electrode is placed in a wet field.

I have never used endodiathermy as an isolated procedure but only as an adjunct in pars plana vitrectomy, where it lets the surgeon perform quite a number of additional tasks such as the coagulation of discrete neovascular stalks, the coagulation of avulsed retinal vessels, and the occlusion of preexisting or inadvertently produced retinal breaks. My experience with endodiathermy as a hemostatic procedure has been disappointing at times, due to the difficulties encountered in locating the bleeding vesel, or to the risks involved in coagulating a vessel overlying the disc.

CHAPTER 10

DIABETIC RETINOPATHY AND PREGNANCY

In spite of some assertions to the contrary, it would seem that retinopathy only rarely makes its first appearance in diabetic women during pregnancy, and that when it does it is a result of the natural course of the disease rather than of the pregnancy itself. Beetham (1950) reported on 119 pregnancies in 70 diabetic patients without retinopathy. None of them had any retinal changes appear other than some venous congestion, even though toxemia or nephropathy was present in 27 % of these pregnant women, and calcification of the crural of illiac arteries in 31 % of those cases in which roentgenograms were taken. Hence, one can predict that a woman who enters pregnancy without evidence of diabetic retinopathy will probably not develop retinopathy during the pregnancy.

The risk of progression of existing retinopathy during pregnancy is a different story. The question cannot be dismissed lightly, for while it is true that retinopathy is present in only a minority of diabetic women during their reproductive life — 10 % according to White (1965), 21 % according to Caird *et al.* (1969) — the sheer number of those who do suffer from retinopathy is considerable. Consequently, every practicing ophthalmologist must expect to be faced sooner or later with the problem of a diabetic woman who is pregnant or who needs counsel about the risks of becoming pregnant.

It is generally agreed that simple retinopathy shows little, if any, tendency to deteriorate over and above the changes which may be attributed to the mere passage of time. Thus, among the 44 patients (63 pregnancies) studied by Beetham who had a retinopathy of the nonproliferative type, eight showed definite progression in the fundus pathology but only four developed proliferative retinopathy. White (1965), on the other hand, has never seen the manifestations of benign retinopathy progress to malignant changes.

By contrast, in cases with malignant or proliferative forms of retinopathy there seems to be a definite risk of deterioration during pregnancy. True, the experience of most authors who have reported on the subject is biased by the fact that patients were referred to them because of the presence of ocular symptoms, or because of the authors' well-known interest in the subject. The figures cited by Beetham, who found that the fundus pathology increased in four out of 12 patients (18 pregnancies) with proliferative retinopathy, are suggestive, as are those of White (1965) who found that of 87 pregnant diabetics with proliferative retinopathy ten had hemorrhagic activity during the first three months of pregnancy, and that 11 of these 20 eyes progressed to blindness. Still more conclusive are the data of Okun *et al.* (1971) and those of Martin and Taft (1972). This writer has seen six diabetic women with malignant retinopathy who subsequently became pregnant; in five of them a rapid growth of the neovascular lesions occurred, with massive intraocular hemorrhage in four. The nefarious influence of pregnancy on proliferative retinopathy is further shown by the remarkable decrease in the rate of progression of the retinopathy, or the actual regression, which usually takes place following the termination of pregnancy in those women who had been showing impairment during that time. It is to be pointed out, however, that in some instances the disease continues on a downhill course after delivery.

It is likely that the deterioration shown by the retinopathy in pregnancy depends upon the insulin-antagonistic, diabetogenic effect of the pituitary-like placental (gonodotrophic and galactopoietic) hormones together with progesterone, estrogens, and their androgenic precursors. Moreover, it must be remembered that pituitary activity rises in pregnancy, and that with the progression of pregnancy degradation of insulin by the growing placenta becomes increasingly more effective. Neither the administration of insulin or oral substitutes, the meticulousness of the diet, the regulation on the fluid balance, nor the administration of female sex hormones — which are all essential for the pregnancy to be brought to a successful end — are able to alter the course of diabetic retinopathy, be it benign or malignant.

The influence of the diabetic status on the outcome of pregnancy is nothing short of disastrous, as this is characterized by increased hazards and failures not only in patients with retinopathy, notably proliferative retinopathy, but also in those without evidence of retinopathy even when proper therapy is given. Spontaneous abortion, stillbirth, and early neonatal death all conspire to lower the survival rate. Many diabetic women of childbearing age have had the disease for 20 years or more and, since at least 80 % of the cases of this duration have reached the late stage of vascular sclerosis, it can be assumed that damage to the small blood vessels of the uterine muscle exists. This would explain the high fetal loss rate found in women with retinopathy, inasmuch as the severity of the changes in the retinal arterioles are roughly comparable to those in the peripheral and visceral arterioles.

Among the many causes of that classical accident of obstetrical diabetes, the antepartum intrauterine death, the following should be singled out: (a) pre-eclamptic toxemia, which in diabetes includes only mild hypertension and is accompanied by minimal proteinuria; (b) ketoacidosis; (c) maternal or placental angiopathy; and (d), more rarely, diabetic infantilism (White, 1965). Hydramnios, which is quite common, favors premature rupture of membranes and delivery prior to viability. Development of severe hydramnios despite the use of an adequate diuretic and dietary regimen is an indication for transabdominal amniocentesis. By allowing the pregnancy to proceed, this procedure may let the infant achieve the degree of maturity required for survival (Driscoll and Gillespie, 1965). Fetal causes include developmental faults as well as abnormal fetal and placental growth, the severity of which tend to be in inverse ratio to the duration of diabetes. Edema and macrosomia with the heaviest birth weights are found in patients with prediabetes, chemical diabetes and short-term overt diabetes; whereas longterm diabetics with pan-vascular lesions produce disproportionately small, lean infants (White, 1965).

Neonatal deaths may result from congenital anomalies but are most often due to the respiratory distress syndrome linked with pulmonary hyaline membranes.

From the data in the literature it appears that fertility in women with controlled diabetes is unimpaired today, and that most diabetic women do quite well if under proper obstetric care. Indeed, the maternal survival rate has been estimated at 99.8%. Fetal survival decreases with increasing severity of retinopathy. Thus, 85 % of fetuses survive in diabetic women without retinopathy, 58 % in women with simple retinopathy, and only 19% in women with proliferative retinopathy (White et al., 1956).

If required, simple retinopathy in pregnant women should be treated by photocoagulation, just as it would in any other patient. In the particular case of exudative retinopathy with macular edema, diuretics and a salt-free diet have been said to bring about rapid improvement (Hamilton et al., 1973). Accounts of the management of the malignant variety are few. Hamilton et al. (1973) reported on two patients who developed rapid proliferation of new vessels during pregnancy and

Fig. 10-1. — Right fundus of a 19-year-old female with diabetes of 16 years duration, who until six months previously had shown bilaterally only some diffuse engorgement of the retinal veins and a few scattered microaneurysms but no proliferative changes. The sequence illustrates the rapid increase of the retinopathy under the influence of pregnancy and the dubious value of photocoagulation treatment. a) When four months pregnant, a marked fullness of all branches of the central retinal vein and a veritable *rubeosis retinae* were present. There was no macular edema and visual acuity was 5/5. b) Gross engorgement and beading of veins and marked irregularities of arteries in area 4-5. c) One month later, after extensive argon laser photocoagulation the clinical picture shows no significant change. d) The condition continued to deteriorate as recurrent neovascularization developed over the treated areas. Hence, the patient was submitted to two further sessions of photocoagulation. This picture was taken 24 hours after the third and last session, when over 1,500 burns had been distributed between the disc and the equator (same area as in b). e) Regression occurred only after delivery by cesarean section on the 38th week. This picture was taken two months following delivery. The number of visible new vessels appears drastically reduced, but those that persist present an anarchic course. An epiretinal proliferation of fibrous tissue can be seen above. The macula was unimpaired, except for a few hemorrhages, and vision was 5/10. Note the mottled, largely confluent photocoagulation scars nasally and inferiorly to the disc.

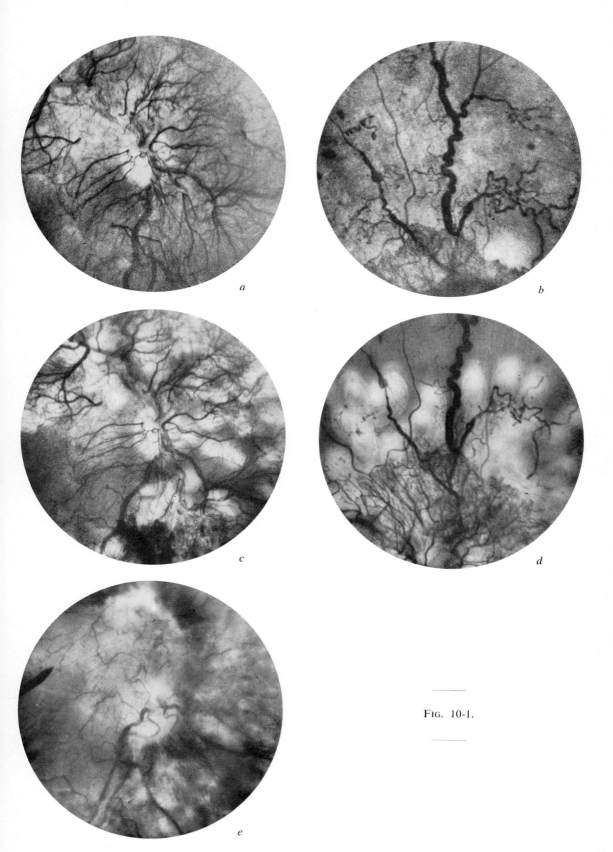

FIG. 10-1.

who were submitted to repeated sessions of photocoagulation, both xenon-arc and argon laser. The response to treatment was not very impressive in the first case, who continued to deteriorate even after delivery, and improved only after pituitary destruction was performed through the implantation of yttrium 90, four and a half months later. In the second case photocoagulation resulted in stabilization, with regression of the retinal lesions after the termination of pregnancy.

In the writer's experience the results of photocoagulation for proliferative diabetic retinopathy in pregnancy have been less fortunate and appear to be unpredictable at best. If permanent in some cases, they are for the most part ephemeral in that an initial regression of the neovascular tissue is succeded by multifocal regrowth, often accompanied by the development of a connective sheet over the photocoagulated areas and by the appearance of fresh vascular tufts and fans peripheral to them (Fig. 10-1).

The case reported by Martin and Taft (1972) where hypophysectomy was performed in the eighth week of pregnancy for rapidly progressing proliferative retinopathy remains unique to this day. The pregnancy proceeded uneventfully, and the patient was delivered of a normal 2930 g. baby on the 37th week by cesarean section.

Regression of the retinopathy commenced after the operation and continued subsequently during a 28-month observation period.

But since the long term mortality and morbidity of pituitary ablation are still uncertain, and its effects on pregnancy imperfectly known, it would seem to me that the logical approach in cases of malignant retinopathy would be to try photocoagulation first, and to put an end to the pregnancy by the 37th week, at which time the infant is large and mature enough to survive. Primary cesarean section should always be preferred since neither the mother, affected by retinopathy and with a propensity to bleed, nor the infant, who is relatively fragile regardless of size or gestational age, will tolerate well a prolonged labor or a difficult operative pelvic delivery (Driscoll and Gillespie, 1965).

To close this section on the relationship between pregnancy and diabetic retinopathy no remark would be more cogent than that of Beetham (1950) who said that all diabetic wives should be encouraged to have their families early in life before many years of diabetes have elapsed and that, in their own best interests, patients presenting a large amount of retinal hemorrhage or with proliferative retinopathy should not be permitted to become pregnant.

CHAPTER 11

CONCLUSIONS

From what has been set forth in this book, it appears that one must concur with Davis (1968) when he says that at best only limited success can be expected from the currently available therapy of diabetic retinopathy. There is adequate evidence now that early diagnosis and good control may delay the onset of the retinopathy, but that once the retinopathy has materialized the most careful control will not reduce its severity or curb its progress.

In the exudative type of background retinopathy the threatment of choice is photocoagulation, either xenon-arc or argon laser, preferably the latter. It can be used freely and repeated at will; it entails practically no risks; and it may succeed in quelling the tendency to retinal edema due to abnormal permeability of the vascular wall and elicit a resorption of the existing circinate deposits, a regression of the venous dilatation with beading, and even an improvement in central vision. The trouble is that the result of photocoagulation is unpredictable in an individual patient. One never knows for sure whether the edema and the multiple microcystoid spaces in the macular region will disappear, whether they will persist unmodified, or whether they will get worse or become complicated by the development of an epiretinal membrane. The trend, however, is toward a slow and substantial amelioration of the retinal lesions with modest visual gains, or without any significant change in vision, so that one may be justified in recommending photocoagulation as the best available treatment against maculopathy.

In the case of the hemorrhagic but nonproliferative form of the disease, the response is much less uncertain since photocoagulation not only provokes a disappearance of the existing microaneurysms and a drastic attenuation of the distended and otherwise altered veins, but usually staves off indefinitely the advent of neovascularization.

In the exudative type of retinopathy a reduced intake of fat should be recommended; in the hemorrhagic type a reduction of elevated blood pressure to lower levels, if not necessarily to normal, should be attempted. In both, the administration of a capillary protector such as calcium dobesilate may be of use.

In the early and intermediate stages of the proliferative type of diabetic retinopathy, photocoagulation should always be used first. But when the response is negative in that the destruction of the new vascular fans cannot be achieved or is followed by a recurrence, and when the extent of the neovascularization — particularly papillovitreal neovascularization — is such that it precludes photocoagulation, the patient should be considered a candidate for pituitary ablation without waiting for him to become worse.

A poor response to photocoagulation should lead us to investigate the 24-hour level of growth hormone. Although this could be done first, of course, my feeling is that even with definitely abnormal values photocoagulation ought to be given a try inasmuch as, for some unknown reason, there are cases that do quite well despite the fact that the somatotrophin levels are consistently elevated, and others that react poorly even if there is no hyperpituitarism and no detectable signs of atherosclerosis.

Anxiety, which springs from the layman's knowledge of the potentialities of diabetic retinopathy, should be grappled with intelligently and strenous physical activity avoided for several reasons.

As a rule, the indications for vitrectomy begin at exactly the same point where those for photocoagulation or hypophysectomy end; it may be used to restore the optical pathway, to relieve traction and to remove the membranes or stalks resulting from the proliferative process. One must not be too enthusiastic in his expectations concerning this procedure, and believe that it can be used without proper consideration or that it will solve unsolvable problems; at the same time one must not leave it until too late. The occurrence of retinal detachment, either rhegmatogenous or nonrhegmatogenous, means that the eye in question may have to be submitted to vitrectomy or to a more conventional, scleral sort of surgery. Such an eye can be expected to get worse with the passage of time and will not improve or even remain unaltered for long. Until recently, vitrectomy for retinal detachment was used only after failure of an external procedure; now it tends to be used as a primary procedure, particularly when traction is strong.

The cure for diabetic retinopathy still lies in the future; it awaits the discovery of the basic underlying biochemical defects and will fall in the province of molecular medicine. For the time being we must continue to resort to the methods described: though ineffective at times, they usually succeed in slowing down the course of the disease and may even achieve some gratifying improvement.

REFERENCES

ADAMS (D. A.), RAND (R. W.), ROTH (N. H.), DASHE (A. M.), GIPSTEIN (R. M.) and HEUSER (G.). — *Diabetes*, 1974, *23*, 698.

ALAERTS (L.) and SLOSSE (J.). — *Bull. Soc. belge ophtal.*, 1957, *3*, 115 (I).

ALMER (L. O.), PANDOLFI (M.) and ØSTERLIN (S.). — *Ophthalmologica* (Basel), 1975, *170*, 353.

AMALRIC (P.). — *Bull. Soc. Ophtal. Fr.*, 1960, *60*, 359.

AMALRIC (P.). — *Act. VII Congr. argent. Oftal.*, 1961, *2*, 181.

AMALRIC (P.). — *Bull. Soc. Ophtal. Fr.*, 1966, *66*, 489.

AMALRIC (P.). — *Ophthalmologica* (Basel), 1967, *154*, 151.

AMALRIC (P.). — *Mod. Probl. Ophthal.*, 1972, *10*, 644.

AMALRIC (P.) and BIAU (C.). — *Arch. Ophtal. (Paris)*, 1967, *27*, 567.

APPLE (D. J.), GOLDBERG (M. F.) and WYHINNY (G.). — *Amer. J. Ophthal*, 1973, *75*, 595.

ARCHER (D.), KRILL (A. E.) and NEWELL (F. W.). — *Trans. ophthal. Soc. U.K.*, 1970, *90*, 677.

ARION (A. F.), CIOLEK (M.), JOSEPH (E.) and POLLIOT (L.). — *Bull. Soc. Ophtal. Fr.*, 1969, *69*, 511.

ASHTON (N.). — *Brit. J. Ophthal.*, 1953, *37*, 282.

ASHTON (N.). — *Fortschr. Augenheilk.*, 1958, *8*, 1.

ASHTON (N.). — *Trans. ophthal. Soc. U.K.*, 1965, *85*, 199.

ASHTON (N.). — *Discussion of Bloodworth*, 1967.

ASHTON (N.). — *Brit. med. Bull.*, 1970, *26*, 143.

ASHTON (N.). — Diabetic retinopathy; some current concepts, *in* Amalric (P.) (Ed.): *Proc. int. Symp. Fluorescein Angiography*, Albi, 1969. Basel, Karger, 1971, 334.

ASHTON (N.). — *Brit. J. Ophthal.*, 1974, *58*, 344.

ASHTON (N.) and CUNHA-VAZ (J. G.). — *Arch. Ophthal.*, 1965, *73*, 211.

BAIRD (J. D.), HUNTER (W. M.) and SMITH (A. W. M.). — *Postgrad. med. J.*, 1973, *49*, 132.

BALLANTYNE (A. J.) and MICHAELSON (I. C.). — *Trans. ophthal. Soc. U.K.*, 1947, *67*, 59.

BALODIMOS (M. C.), REES (S. B.), AIELLO (L. M.), BRADLEY (R. F.) and MARBLE (A.). — Fluorescein photography in proliferative diabetic retinopathy treated by pituitary ablation, *in* GOLDBERG (M. F.) and FINE (S. L.) (Eds.): *Symposium on the Treatment of Diabetic Retinopathy*. Washington, D.C., U.S. Department of Health, Education and Welfare, Public Health Service Publication No. 1890, 1968, 153.

V. BARSEWISCH (B.). — *Klin. Mbl. Augenheilk.*, 1971, *159*, 742.

BEAUMONT (P.) and HOLLOWS (F. C.). — *Lancet*, 1972, *1*, 419.

BEAVEN (D. W.), NELSON (D. H.), RENOLD (A. E.) and THORN (G. W.) — *New Engl. J. Med.*, 1959, *261*, 443.

BECKER (B.). — *Trans. Amer. Acad. Ophthal.*, 1971, *75*, 239.

BECKER (B.), BRESNICK (G.), CHEVRETTE (L.), KOLKER (A. E.), OAKS (M. C.) and CIBIS (A.). — *Arch. Ophthal.*, 1966, *76*, 477.

BEETHAM (W. P.). — *Trans. Amer. ophthal. Soc.*, 1950, *48*, 205.

BEETHAM (W. P.). — *Brit. J. Ophthal.*, 1963, *47*, 611.

BEETHAM (W. P.), AIELLO (L. M.), BALODIMOS (M. C.) and KONCZ (L.). — *Arch. Ophthal.*, 1970, *83*, 261.

BERKOW (J. W), SHUGARMAN (R. G.), MAUMENEE (A. E.) and PATZ (A.). — *J. Amer. med. Ass.*, 1965, *193*, 867.

BISANTIS (C.). — *Boll. Oculist.*, 1971, *50*, 153.

BLOODWORTH (J. M. B.). — *Diabetes*, 1962, *11*, 1.

BLOODWORTH (J. M. B.). — *Diabetes*, 1963, *12*, 99.

BLOODWORTH (J. M. B.). — Fine structure of retina in human and canine diabetes mellitus, *in* KIMURA (S. J.) and CAYGILL (W. M.) (Eds.): *Vascular Complications of Diabetes Mellitus with Special Emphasis on Microangiopathy of the Eye*. Saint Louis, Mosby, 1967, 73.

BLOODWORTH (J. M. B.) and ENGERMAN (R. L.). — *Diabetes*, 1973, *22*, 290, suppl. 1.

BLOODWORTH (J. M. B.) and MOLITOR (D. L.). — *Invest. Ophthal.*, 1965, *4*, 1037.

BONIUK (I.), OKUN (E.) and JOHNSTON (G. P.). — *Mod. Probl. Ophthal.*, 1972, *10*, 341.

BONNET (M.). — *Conf. lyon. Ophtal.*, 1972, *116*, 3.

BONNET (M.) and PINGAULT (C.). — *Bull. Soc. Ophtal. Fr.,* 1971, *71,* 687.

BORGMANN (H.), REUSCHER (A.) and MIES (S.). — *Klin. Mbl. Augenheilk.,* 1974, *164,* 752.

BOUZAS (A. G.), GRAGOUDAS (E. S.), BALODIMOS (M. C.), BRINEGAR (C. H.) and AIELLO (L. M.). — *Arch. Ophthal.,* 1971, *85,* 423.

BRADLEY (R. F.) and RAMOS (G.). — The eyes and diabetes, *in* MARBLE (A.), WHITE (P.), BRADLEY (R. F.) and KRALL (L. P.) (Eds.): *Joslin's Diabetes Mellitus.* Philadelphia Lea & Febiger 11th ed., 1971, 478.

BRADLEY (R. F.) and REES (S. B.). — Surgical pituitary ablation for diabetic retinopathy, *in* GOLDBERG (M. F.) and FINE (S. L.) (Eds.): *Symposium on the Treatment of Diabetic Retinopathy.* Washington, D.C., U.S. Department of Health, Education and Welfare, Public Health Service Publication No. 1890, 1968, 171.

BRAZEAU (P.), RIVIER (J.), VALE (W.) and GUILLEMIN (R.). — *Endocrinology,* 1974, *94,* 184.

BRAZEAU (P.), VALE (W.), BURGUS (R.), LING (N.), BUTCHER (M.), RIVIER (J.) and GUILLEMIN (R.). — *Science,* 1973, *179,* 77.

BRESNICK (G. H.), De VENECIA (G.), MYERS (F. L.), HARRIS (J. A.) and DAVIS (M. D.). — *Arch. Ophthal.,* 1975, *93,* 1300.

BRESNICK (G. H.), MYERS (F. L.), DE VENECIA (G.) and DAVIS (M. D.). — *Vitreous pathology in proliferative diabetic retinopathy. To be published,* 1975.

BRONSON (N. R.). — *J. clin. Ultrasound,* 1973, *1,* 102.

BRONSON (N. R.). — *Amer. J. Ophthal.,* 1974, *77,* 181.

BRYFOGLE (J. W.) and BRADLEY (R. F.). — *Diabetes,* 1957, *6,* 159.

BURDITT (A. F.), CAIRD (F. I.) and DRAPER (G. J.). — *Quart. J. Med.,* 1968, *37,* 303.

CAIRD (F. I.). — *Diabetes,* 1967, *16,* 502.

CAIRD (F. I). — Control of diabetes and diabetic retinopathy, *in* GOLDBERG (M. F.) and FINE (S. L.) (Eds.): *Symposium on the Treatment of Diabetic Retinopathy.* Washington, D.C., U.S. Department of Health, Education and Welfare, Public Health Service Publication No. 1890, 1968, 107.

CAIRD (F. I.) and GARRET (C. J.). — *Proc. roy. Soc. Med.,* 1962, *55,* 477.

CAIRD (F. I.) and GARRET (C. J.). — *Diabetes,* 1963, *12,* 389.

CAIRD (F. I.), PIRIE (A.) and RAMSELL (T. G.). — *Diabetes and the Eye,* Oxford and Edinburgh, Blackwell, 1968, *passim.*

CHERVIN (M.), De VECCHI (H. P.) and VACARO (G.). — *Arch. Oftal. B. Aires,* 1973, *48,* 337.

CLEASBY (G. W.) — Photocoagulation therapy of diabetic retinopathy, *in* GOLDBERG (M. F.) and FINE (S. L.) (Eds): *Symposium on the Treatment of Diabetic Retinopathy.* Washington, D.C., U.S. Depart-

ment of Health, Education and Welfare, Public Health Service Publication No. 1890, 1968, 465.

COGAN (D. G.). — *New Engl. J. Med.,* 1964, *270,* 787.

COGAN (D. G.) and KUWABARA (T.). — Ocular microangiopathy in diabetes, *in* KIMURA (S. J.) and CAYGILL (W. M.) (Eds.): *Vascular Complications of Diabetes Mellitus, with Special Emphasis on Microangiopathy of the Eye.* Saint Louis, Mosby, 1967, 53.

COGAN (D. G.), TOUSSAINT (M. D.) and KUWABARA (T.). — *Arch. Ophthal.,* 1961, *66,* 366.

COLEMAN (D. J.). — *Amer. J. Ophthal.,* 1972, *73,* 501.

COLEMAN (D. J.) and FRANZEN (L. A.). — *Arch. Ophthal.,* 1974, *92,* 375.

CONSTAM (G. R.). — *Helv. med. Acta,* 1965, *32,* 287.

CRISTIANSSON (J.). — *Acta Ophthal.* (Kbh.), 1965, *43,* 224.

CRISTINI (G.) and TOLOMELLI (E.). — *Arch. Pat. Clin. med.,* 1947, *25,* 275.

CULLEN (J. F.), IRELAND (J. T.) and OLIVER (M. F.). — *Trans. ophthal. Soc. U.K.,* 1964, *84,* 281.

CULLEN (J. F.), TOWN (S. M.) and CAMPBELL (C. J.). — *Trans ophthal. Soc. U.K.,* 1974, *94,* 554.

CUNHA-VAZ (J. G.) — *Trans. ophthal. Soc. U.K.,* 1972, *92,* 111.

CUNHA-VAZ (J. G.), SHAKIB (M.) and ASHTON (N.). — *Brit. J. Ophthal.,* 1966, *50,* 441.

DAMASKE (M. M.), COHEN (D. N.), GUTMAN (F. A.) and SCHUMACHER (O. P.). — *J. pediat. Ophthal.,* 1975, *12,* 16.

DAVANGER (M.). — *Acta ophtal* (Kbh.), 1961, *39,* 1.

DAVIS (M. D.). — *Arch. Ophthal.,* 1965, *74,* 741.

DAVIS (M. D.). — Natural course of diabetic retinopathy, *in* KIMURA (S. J.) and CAYGILL (W. M.) (Eds.): *Vascular Complications of Diabetes Mellitus with Special Emphasis on Microangiopathy of the Eye.* Saint Louis, Mosby, 1967, 139.

DAVIS (M. D.). — *Trans. Amer. Acad. Ophthal.,* 1968, *72,* 237.

DAVIS (M. D.). — *Modification of Airlie House classification of diabetic retinopathy.* Instruction sheet supplied on request by the University of Wisconsin Department of Ophthalmology, 1972.

DAVIS (M. D.), MYERS (F. L.), ENGERMANN (R. L.), De VENECIA (G.) and BRESNIEK (G. H.). — *Proc. 8th. Congr. int. Diabetes Fed.,* Brussels, 1973, 439.

DAVIS (M. D.), NORTON (E. W. D.) and MYERS (F. L.). — The Airlie classification of diabetic retinopathy, *in* GOLDBERG (M. F.) and FINE (S. L.) (Eds.): *Symposium on the Treatment of Diabetic Retinopathy.* Washington, D. C., U.S. Department of Health, Education and Welfare, Public Health Service Publication no. 1890, 1968, 7.

DECKERT (T.), SIMONSEN (S. E.) and POULSEN (J. E.). — Diabetes, 1967, *16,* 728.

DELLAPORTA (A.). — *Klin. Mbl. Augenheilk,* 1951, *118,* 337.

DELLAPORTA (A.) and DECLERCQ (S. D.). — *Trans. Amer. Acad. Ophthal.,* 1973, *77,* 27.

DOBBIE (J. G.), KWAN (H. C.), COLWELL (J. A.) and SUWANWELA (N.). — *Trans. Amer. Acad. Ophthal.,* 1973, *77,* 43.

DOBBIE (J. G.), KWAN (H. C.), COLWELL (J. A.) and SUWANWELA (N.). — *Arch. Ophthal.* 1974, *91,* 107.

DOBREE (J. H.). — *Brit. J. Ophthal.,* 1964*a, 48,* 637.

DOBREE (J. H.). — *Trans. ophthal. Soc. U.K.,* 1964*b, 84,* 521.

DOBREE (J. H.). — *Brit. J. Opthal.,* 1970*a,* 54, 1.

DOBREE (J. H.). — *Trans. ophthal. Soc. U.K.,* 1970*b, 90,* 669.

DOBREE (J. H.) and TAYLOR (E.). — *Trans. ophthal. Soc. U.K.,* 1968, *88,* 313.

DOBREE (J. H.) and TAYLOR (E.). — *Brit. J. Ophthal.,* 1973, *57,* 73.

DODEN (W.). — *Klin. Mbl. Augenheilk.,* 1974, *164,* 441.

DOLLERY (C. T.). — *Trans. ophthal. Soc. U.K.,* 1973, *93,* 513.

DOLLERY (C. T.) and OAKLEY (N. W.). — *Diabetes,* 1965, *14,* 121.

DOLLERY (C. T.) and KOHNER (E. M.). — *Proc. 8th. Congr. int. Diabetes Fed.,* Brussels, 1973, 443.

DOUVAS (N. G.). — *Trans. Amer. Acad. Ophthal.,* 1973, *77,* 792.

DOUVAS (N. G.). — *Mod. Probl. Ophthal.,* 1975, *15,* 253.

DRISCOLL (J. J.) and GILLESPIE (L.). — *Med. Clin. N. Amer.,* 1965, *49,* 1025.

DUANE (T. D.). — *Amer. J. Opthhal.,* 1971, *71,* 286.

DUFOUR (R.). — *Mod. Probl. Ophthal.,* 1967, *5,* 93.

DUKE-ELDER (S.) and DOBREE (J. H.). — Diseases af the retina, *in* DUKE-ELDER (S.): *System of Ophthalmology.* London, Kimpton, 1967, *10,* 408.

DUNCAN (L. J. P.), NOLAN (J.), IRELAND (J. T.), CULLEN (J. F.), CLARKE (B. F.) and OLIVER (M. F.). — *Diabetes,* 1968, *17,* 458.

EISALO (A.) and RAITTA (C.). — *Eye, Ear, Nose Thr. Monthly,* 1971, *50,* 447.

EISNER (G.). — *Biomicroscopy of the Peripheral Fundus.* Berlin & New York, Springer, 1973, 45.

ENTMACHER (P. S.) and MARKS (H. H.). — *Diabetes,* 1964, *14,* 212.

ERNEST (I.), LINNER (M. E.) and SVANBORG (A.). — *Amer. J. Med.,* 1965, *39,* 594.

ESMANN (V.), JENSEN (H. J.) and LUNDBAEK (K.). — *Acta med. scand.,* 1963, *174,* 99.

FANKHAUSER (F.) and LOTMAR (W.). — *Klin. Mbl. Augenheilk.,* 1972, *160,* 218.

FANKHAUSER (F.), LOTMAR (W.) and ROULIER (A.). — *Graefes Arch. klin. exp. Ophthal.,* 1972*a, 183,* 334.

FANKHAUSER (F.), LOTMAR (W.) and ROULIER (A.). — *Graefes Arch. klin. exp. Ophthal.,* 1972*b, 184,* 111.

FERRER (O.). — Retinal circulation time in the diabetic patient, *in* SHIMIZU (K.) (Ed.): *Fluorescein Angiography.* Tokyo, Igaku Shoin, 1974, 23.

FIELD (R. A.). — *Trans. Amer. Acad. Ophthal.,* 1968, *72,* 241.

FINLEY (J. K.). — *Angiology,* 1961, *12,* 127.

FINLEY (J. K.) and WEAVER (H. S. Jr.). — *Amer. J. Ophthal.,* 1960, *50,* 483.

FISCHER (F.). — *Graefes Arch. Ophthal.,* 1961, *163,* 397.

FISCHER (F.). — *Graefes Arch. Ophthal.,* 1963, *166,* 220.

FISCHER (F.). — *Graefes Arch. Ophthal.,* 1964, *167,* 607.

FISCHER (F.). — *Klin. Mbl. Augenheilk.,* 1972, *160,* 320.

FRANCESCHETTI (A.). — *Amer. J. Ophthal.,* 1955, *39,* 189.

FRANK (R. N.). — *Arch. Ophthal.,* 1975, *93,* 591.

FRASER (R.). — Treatment of retinopathy by pituitary ablation, *in* DUNCAN (L. J. P.) (Ed.): *Diabetes Mellitus.* Edinburgh, University Press, 1966, 177.

FRASER (R.), KOHNER (E. M.), JOPLIN (G. F.), DOYLE (F. H.), HAMILTON (A. M.) and BLACH (R. K.). — *Proc. 8th. Congr. int. Diabetes Fed.,* Brussels, 1973, 431.

FREYLER (H.). — *Klin. Mbl. Augenheilk.,* 1974, *164,* 760.

FREYLER (H.) and NICHORLIS (S.). — *Klin. Mbl. Augenheilk.,* 1974, *165,* 594.

FREYLER (H.) and SEHORST (W.). — *Klin. Mbl. Augenheilk.,* 1974, *164,* 246.

FREZZOTI (R.), BARDELLI (A. M.), LENTI (G.) and PAGANO (G.). — *Boll. Oculist.* 1952, *51,* 219.

FULLER (D. G.) and KNJGHTON (R. W.). — *Amer. J. Ophthal.,* 1975, *80,* 214.

GARNER (A.) and ASHTON (N.). — *Trans. ophthal. Soc. U.K.,* 1972, *92,* 101.

GAVEY (C. J.). — *Brit. J. Ophthal.,* 1966, *50,* 689.

GAY (A. J.) and ROSENBAUM (A. L.). — *Arch. Ophthal.,* 1966, *75,* 758.

GERRITZEN (F. M.). — *Diabetes,* 1973, *22,* 122.

GILLS (J. P., Jr.) and ANDERSON (W. B., Jr.). — *Arch. inter. Med.,* 1969, *123,* 626.

GODLOWSKI (Z.), GAZDA (M.) and WITHERS (B. T.). — *Laryngoscope* (St. Louis) 1961, *81,* 1337.

GOLDBERG (M. F.) and FINE (S. L.) (Eds.). — *Symposium on the Treatment of Diabetic Retinopathy.* Washington, D.C., U.S. Department of Health, Education and Welfare, Public Health Publication no. 1890, 1968, p. XXI.

GRAFE (E.). — *Klin. Mbl. Augenheilk.,* 1923, *69,* 841.

GRAFE (E.). — *Ber. dtsch. ophthal. Ges.,* 1924, *44,* 53.

GRAHAM (P. A.). — *Brit. J. Ophthal.*, 1972, *56*, 223.

GUINAN (P.). — *Brit. J. Ophthal.*, 1967, *51*, 289.

GUINAN (P.). — *Trans. ophthal. Soc. U.K.*, 1968, *88*, 741.

HAM (W. T.)., WIESINGER (H.), SCHMIDT (F. H.), WILLIAMS (R. C.), RUFFIN (R. S.), SHAFFER (M. C.) and GUERRY (D.). — *Amer J. Ophthal.*, 1958, *46*, 700.

HAMILTON (A. M.), KOHNER (E. M.), BLACH (R. K.) and BOWBYES (J. A.). — *Trans. ophthal. Soc. U.K.*, 1973, *93*, 571.

HARDIN (R. C.), JACKSON (R. L.), JOHNSTON (T. L.) and KELLY (H. G.). — *Diabetes*, 1956, *5*, 397.

HARDY (J.), PANISSET (A.), MARCHILDON (A.) and LENTHIER (A.). — Transphenoidal microsurgical selective anterior pituitary ablation: a pathophysiological investigation of diabetic retinopathy, *in* GOLDBERG (M. F.) and FINE (S. L.) (Eds.): *Symposium on the Treatment of Diabetic Retinopathy.* Washington, D.C., U.S. Department of Health, Education and Welfare, Public Health Service Publication no. 1890, 1968, 235.

HARROLD (B. P.), MARMION (V. J.) and GOUGH (K. R.). — *Diabetes*, 1969, *18*, 285.

HATFIELD (R. E.), GASTINEAU (C. F.) and RUCKER (C. W.). — *Proc. Mayo Clin.*, 1962, *37*, 513.

HEATH (H.), BRIDGEN (W. D.), CANEVER (J. D.), POLLOCK (J.), HUNTER (P. R.), KELSEY (J.) and BLOOM (A.). — *Diabetologia*, 1971, *7*, 308.

HENKIND (P.). — *Proc. 8th. Congr. int. Diabetes Fed.*, Brussels, 1973, 448.

HILL (D. W.). — *Trans. ophthal. Soc. U.K.* 1972, *92*, 125.

HOUSSAY (B. A.) and BIASOTTI (A.). — *Rev. Soc. argent. Biol.*, 1930, *6*, 251.

HOUSSAY (B. A.) and BIASOTTI (A.). — *Pflügers Arch. ges. Physiol.*, 1931, *227*, 664.

HOUSSAY (B. A.) and RODRIGUEZ (R. R.). — *Endocrinology*, 1953, *53*, 114.

HOUTSMULLER (A. J.). — *Ophthalmologica (Basel)*, 1968, *156*, 2.

HOUTSMULLER (A. J.). — *Klin. Mbl. Augenheilk.*, 1972, *160*, 521.

HUNTER (P. R.), COTTON (S. G.), KELSEY (J. H.) and BLOOM (A.). — *Brit. med. J.*, 1967, *2*, 651.

IGERSHEIMER (J.). — *Arch. Ophthal.*, 1944, *32*, 50.

IKKOS (D.) and LUFT (R.). — *Lancet*, 1960, *2*, 897.

IRVINE (A. R.) and NORTON (E. W. D.). — *Amer. J. Ophthal.*, 1971, *71*, 437.

JACK (R. L.), HUTTON (W. L.) and MACHEMER (R.). — *Amer. J. Ophthal.*, 1974, *78*, 265.

JAIN (I. S.), LUTHRA (C. L.) and DAS (T.). — *Arch. Ophthal.*, 1967, *77*, 59.

JAMES (W. A.) and L'ESPERANCE (F. A.). — *Amer. J. Ophthal.*, 1974, *78*, 939.

JOHANSEN (K.) and HANSEN (A. P.). — *Brit. med. J.*, 1969, *2*, 356.

JOPLIN (G. F.), FRASER (T. R.), HILL (D. W.), OAKLEY (N. W.), SCOTT (D.) and DOYLE (F.). — *Quart. J. Med.*, 1965, *35*, 443.

JOPLIN (G. F.), OAKLEY (N.), KOHNER (E. M.), HILL (D. W.) and FRASER (T. R.). — Diabetologia, 1967, *3*, 406.

KAHN (H. A.) and BRADLEY (R. F.). — *Brit. J. Ophthal.*, 1975, *59*, 345.

KAHN (H. A.) and HILLER (R.). — *Amer. J. Ophthal.*, 1974, *78*, 58.

KASNER (D.), MILLER (G. R.), TAYLOR (W. H.), SEVER (R. J.) and NORTON (E. W. D.). — *Trans. Amer. Acad. Ophthal.*, 1968, *72*, 410.

KEARNS (T. P.) and HOLLENHORST (R. W.). — *Proc. Mayo Clin.*, 1963, *38*, 304.

KEEN (A.) and SMITH (R.). — *Lancet*, 1959, *1*, 849.

KEENEY (A. H.) and MODY (M. V.). — *Arch. Ophthal.*, 1955, *54*, 665.

KEMPNER (W.), PESCHEL (R. L.) and SCHLAYER (C.). — *Postgrad. Med.*, 1958, *24*, 359.

KING (R. C.), DOBREE (J. H.), KOK (D'A.), FOULDS (W. S.) and DANGERFIELD (W. G.). — *Brit. J. Ophthal.*, 1963, *47*, 666.

KLÖTI (R.). — *Graefes Arch. klin. exp. Ophthal.*, 1973, *187*, 161.

KLÖTI (R.). — *Graefes Arch. klin. exp. Ophthal.*, 1974, *189*, 125.

KLÖTI (R.). — *Vitrectomy, a pars plana approach. To be published*, 1974.

KNOPF (R. F.), FAJANS (S. S.), PEK (S.) and CONN (J. W.). — *Diabetes*, 1972, *21*, 322.

KNOWLES (H. C., Jr.). — The control of diabetes mellitus and the progression of retinopathy, *in* GOLDBERG (M. F.) and FINE (S. L.) (Eds.): *Symposium on the Treatment of Diabetic Retinopathy.* Washington, D.C., U.S. Department of Health, Education and Welfare, Public Health Service Publication no. 1890, 1968a, 115.

KNOWLES (H. C., Jr.). — Summary of papers on relationship of retinopathy to metabolic control, *in* GOLDBERG (M. F.) and FINE (S. L.) (Eds.): *Symposium on the Treatment of Diabetic Retinopathy.* Washington, D.C., Department of Health, Education and Welfare, Public Health Publication no. 1890, 1968b, 129.

KOHNER (E. N.) and DOLLERY (C. T.). — *Europ. J. clin. Invest.*, 1970, *1*, 167.

KOHNER (E. M.), DOLLERY (C. T.), PATERSON (J. W.) and OAKLEY (N. W.). — *Diabetes*, 1967, *16*, 1.

KOHNER (E. M.), FRASER (T. R.), JOPLIN (G. F.) and OAKLEY (N. W.). — The effect of diabetic control on diabetic retinopathy, *in* GOLDBERG (M. F.) and FINE (S. L.) (Eds.): *Symposium on the Treatment of Diabetic Retinopathy.* Washington, D.C., U.S. Department of Health, Education and Welfare,

Public Health Service Publication no. 1890, 1968, 119.

KOHNER (E. M.), HAMILTON (A. M.), JOPLIN (G. F.) and FRASER (T. R.). — *Diabetes*, 1976, *25*, 104.

KOHNER (E. M.), JOPLIN (G. F.), BLACH (R. K.), CHENG (H.) and FRASER (T. R.). — *Trans. ophthal. Soc. U.K.*, 1972, *92*, 79.

KOLODNY (H. D.), SHERMAN (L.), SINGH (A.), FUN (S.) and BENJAMIN (F.). — *New Engl. J. Med.*, 1971, *284*, 819.

KUWABARA (T.) and COGAN (D. G.). — *Arch. Ophthal.*, 1973, *69*, 492.

LAQUA (H.). — *Pre- and subretinal gliosis*, 1974. To be published.

LARSEN (H. W.). — *Acta ophthal.* (Kbh.), 1959, *37*, 531.

LEE (P. F.), MCMEEL (J. W.), SCHEPENS (C. L.) and FIELD (R. A.). — *Amer. J. Ophthal.* 1966, *62*, 207.

LERCHE (W.) and BEEGER (R.). — *Ber. dtsch. ophthal. Ges.*, 1972, *72*, 216.

L'ESPERANCE (F. A., Jr.). — *Trans. Amer. ophthal. Soc.*, 1968, *66*, 826.

L'ESPERANCE (F. A., Jr.). — *Trans. Amer. Acad. Ophthal.*, 1969, *73*, 1077.

L'ESPERANCE (F. A.). — *Trans. Amer. Acad. Ophthal.*, 1973, *77*, 6,

L'ESPERANCE (F. A., Jr.), LABUDA (E. F.) and JOHNSON (A. M.). — *Brit. J. Ophthal.* 1969, *53*, 310.

LEUENBERGER (P. M.), BEAUCHEMIN (M. L.) and BABEL (J.). — *Arch. Ophtal. (Paris)*, 1974, *34*, 289.

LIMON (S.), HAUT (J.) and SALVODELLI (M.). — *Arch. Ophtal. (Paris)*, 1973, *33*, 593.

LITTLE (H. L.). — Argon laser therapy of diabetic retinopathy *in* FRANÇOIS, (J.) (Ed.): *Symposium on Light Coagulation*. The Hague, Junk, 1973*b*, 77.

LITTLE (H. L.). — Preventing complications in argon laser retina photocoagulation, *in* FRANÇOIS (J.) (Ed.): *Symposium on Light Coagulation*. The Hague, Junk, 1973*b*, 87.

LITTLE (H. L.) and ZWENG (H. C.). — *Trans. Pacif. Cst. oto-ophthal. Soc.*, 1971, *52*, 115.

LITTLE (H. L.) and ZWENG (H. C.). — *Trans. Amer. Acad. Ophthal.*, in press.

LITTLE (H. L.), ZWENG (H. C.) and PEABODY (R. R.). — *Trans. Amer. Acad. Ophthal.*, 1970, *74*, 85.

LIUZZI (A.), CHIODINI (P. G.), BOTALLA (L.) and SILVESTRINI (F.). — *Ann. Endocr. (Paris)*, 1972, 33, 426.

LOURRIE (H.), MOSES (A.) and LLOYD (C.). — *New Engl. J. Med.*, 1962, *267*, 924.

LUFT (R.) and GUILLEMIN (R.). — *Diabetes*, 1974, *23*, 783.

LUFT (R.), OLIVECRONA (H.), IKKOS (D.), KORNERUP (T.) and LJUNGGREN (H.). — *Brit. med. J.*, 1955*b*, 2, 752.

LUFT (R.), OLIVECRONA (H.) and SJÖGREN (B.). — *Nord. Med.*, 1952, *47*, 351.

LUFT (R.), OLIVECRONA (H.) and SJÖGREN (B.). — *J. clin. Endocr.*, 1955*a*, *15*, 391.

LUNDBAEK (K.), CHRISTENSEN (N. J.), JENSEN (V. A.), JOHANSEN (K.), OLSEN (T. S.), HANSEN (A. P.), ORSKOV (H.) and OSTERBY (R.). — *Lancet*, 1970, *2*, 131.

LUNDBAEK (K.), CHRISTENSEN (N. J.), JENSEN (V. A.), JOHANSEN (K.), OLSEN (T. S.), HANSEN (A. P.), ORSKOV (H.) and OSTERBY (R.). — *Dan. med. Bull.*, 1971, *18*, 1.

LUNDBAEK (K.), MALMROS (R.), ANDERSEN (H. C.), RASMUSSEN (H. H.), BRUNTSE (E.), MADSEN (P. H.) and JENSEN (V. A.). — Hypophysectomy for diabetic angiopathy: a controlled clinical trial, *in* GOLDBERG (M. F.) and FINE (S. L.) (Eds.): *Symposium on the Treatment of Diabetic Retinopathy*. Washington, D.C., U.S. Department of Health, Education and Welfare, Public Health Service Publication no. 1890, 1968, 291.

LYALL (A.) and INNES (J. A.). — *Lancet*, 1935, *1*, 318.

MACHEMER (R.). — *Amer. J. Ophthal.*, 1972, *74*, 1022.

MACHEMER (R.). — *Trans. Amer. Acad. Ophthal.*, 1973*a*, *77*, 198.

MACHEMER (R.). — *Klin. Mbl. Augenheilk.*, 1973*b*, *162*, 199.

MACHEMER (R.). — *Arch. Ophthal.*, 1974*a*, *92*, 402.

MACHEMER (R.). — *Arch. Ophthal.*, 1974*b*, *92*, 407.

MACHEMER (R.), BUETTNER (H.), NORTON (E.W.D.) and PAREL (J. M.). — *Trans. Amer. Acad. Ophthal.*, 1971, *75*, 813.

MACHEMER (R.) and NORTON (E. W. D.). — *Amer. J. Ophthal.*, 1972*a*, *74*, 1034.

MACHEMER (R.) and NORTON (E. W. D.). — *Mod. Probl. Ophthal.*, 1972*b*, *10*, 178.

MACHEMER (R.), PAREL (J. M.) and BUETTNER (H.). — *Amer. J. Ophthal.*, 1972, *73*, 1.

MACHEMER (R.), PAREL (J. M.) and NORTON (E. W. D.). — *Trans. Amer. Acad. Ophthal.*, 1972, *76*, 462.

MACKENZIE (W.). — *Ophthal. Hosp. Rep.*, 1877, *9*, 134.

MARKS (H. H.), KRALL (L. P.) and WHITE (P.). — Epidemiology and detection of diabetes, *in* MARBLE (A.), WHITE (P.), BRADLEY (R. F.) and KRALL (L. P.) (Eds): *Joslin's Diabetes Mellitus*. Philadelphia, Lea & Febiger, 11th ed., 1971, 10.

MARRÉ (E.) and MARRÉ (M.). — *Klin. Mbl. Augenheilk.*, 1968, *153*, 396.

MARTIN (F. I. R.) and TAFT (P.). — *Diabetes*, 1972, *21*, 972.

MAUMENEE (A. E.). — *Trans. ophthal. Soc. U.K.*, 1968, *88*, 529.

MAUTNER (W.). — *Klin. Mbl. Augenheilk.*, 1974, *164*, 807.

MCCULLAGH (E. P.). — *Diabetes*, 1956, *5*, 223.

MCMEEL (J. W.). — *Trans. Amer. ophthal. Soc.*, 1971, *69*, 440.

MEHNERT (H.). — *Dtsch. med. Wschr.*, 1969, *94*, 42.

MEISSNER (C.), THUM (Ch.), BEISCHER (W.), WINKLER (G.), SCHRÖDER (K. E.) and PFEIFER (E. F.). — *Diabetes*, 1975, *24*, 988.

MERIMEE (T. J.), SIPERSTEIN (M. D.), HALL (J. D.) and FINEBERG (S. E.). — *J. clin. Invest.*, 1970, *49*, 2161.

MEYER-SCHWICKERATH (G.). — *Lichtkoagulation.* Stuttgart, Enke, 1959, 61.

MEYER-SCHWICKERATH (G.) and SCHOTT (K.) — *Klin. Mbl. Augenheilk.*, 1968, *153*, 173.

MOONEY (A. J.). — *Brit. J. Ophthal.*, 1963, *47*, 513.

MOTTA (G.), BOLES CARENINI (B.), PIRODDA (A.) and ORZALESI (N.). — *Ann. Ottal.* 1971, *97*, 245.

NEMETH (B.), HUDOMEL (J.) and FARKAS (A.). — *Ophthalmologica* (Basel), 1975, *170*, 434.

NETTLESHIP (E.). — *Trans. ophthal. Soc. U.K.*, 1888, *8*, 161.

OAKLEY (N. W.), HILL (D. W.), JOPLIN (G. F.), KOHNER (E. M.) and FRASER (T. R.). — *Diabetologia*, 1967, *3*, 402.

OAKLEY (N. W.), JOPLIN (G. F.), KOHNER (E. M.) and FRASER (T. R.). — The treatment of diabetic retinopathy by pituitary implantation, *in* GOLDBERG (M. F.) and FINE (S. L.) (Eds.): *Symposium on the Treatment of Diabetic Retinopathy.* Washington, D.C., U.S. Department of Health, Education and Welfare, Public Health Service Publication no. 1890, 1968, 317.

OFFRET (G.) and GUYOT (C.). — *Arch. Ophtal. (Paris)*, 1972, *32*, 241.

OFFRET (G.), POULIQUEN (Y.) and GUYOT (C.). — *Atherogenesis.* Amsterdam, Excerpta Medica, International Congress Series no. 201, 1969, 189.

OKUN (E.). — *Trans. Amer. Acad. Ophthal.*, 1968, *72*, 246.

OKUN (E.) and CIBIS (P.). — *Arch. Ophthal.*, 1966, *75*, 337.

OKUN (E.) and FUNG (W. E.). — Therapy of diabetic retinal detachment, *in* Symposium on Retina and Retinal Surgery, *Trans. New Orleans Acad. Ophthal.*, St. Louis, Mosby, 1969, 319.

OKUN (E.), JOHNSTON (G. P.) and BONIUK (I.). — *Management of Diabetic Retinopathy.* St. Louis, Mosby, 1971, *passim*.

OLIVELLA (A.). — *Mod. Probl. Ophthal.*, 1972, *10*, 325.

OOSTERHUIS (J. A.), LOEWER-SIEGER (D. H.) and VAN GOOL (J.). — *Acta ophthal.* (Kbh), 1963, *41*, 354.

ORSKOV (H.), THOMSEN (H. G.) and YDE (H.). — *Nature*, 1968, *219*, 193.

PANDOLFI (M.), ALMÉR (L. O.) and HOLMBERG (L.). — *Acta Ophthal.* (Kbh.), 1974, *52*, 823.

PANISSET (A.), KOHNER (E. M.), CHENG (H.) and FRASER (T. R.). — *Diabetes, 20*, 1971, 284.

PANNARALE (M. R.). — *Mod. Probl. Ophthal.*, 1969, *8*, 511.

PATZ (A.). — *Surv. Ophthal.*, 1972, *16*, 249.

PATZ (A.) and BERKOW (J. W.). — *Trans. Amer. Acad. Ophthal.*, 1968, *72*, 253.

PAZ-GUEVARA (A.), HAU (T. H.) and WHITE (P.). — *Diabetes*, 1974, *23*, 357.

PEYMAN (G. A.), DAILY (M. J.) and ERICSON (E. S.). — *Amer J. Ophthal.*, 1973, *75*, 774.

PEYMAN (G. A.), SPITZNAS (M.) and STRAATSMA (B. R.). — *Invest. Ophthal.*, *10*, 1971, 489.

PLANGE (H.). — *Graefes Arch. klin. exp. Ophthal.*, 1971, *183*, 210.

PORTSMANN (W.) and WIESE (J.). — *Klin. Mbl. Augenheilk.*, 1954, *125*, 336.

POULSEN (J. E.). — *Diabetes*, 1953, *2*, 7.

POULSEN (J. E.). — *Diabetes*, 1966, *15*, 3.

POWELL (E. D. U.), FRANTZ (A. G.), RABKIN (M. T.) and FIELD (R. A.). — *New Engl. J. Med.*, 1966, *275*, 922.

PRICE (J.), STAUFFER (H. H.), HOGAN (W. D.) and LAWRENCE (J. H.). — *Brit. J. Ophthal.*, 1972, *56*, 21.

RAY (B. S.), PAZIANOS (A. G.), GREENBERG (E.), PERETZ (W. L.) and MCLELAN (J. M.. — *J. Amer. med. Ass.*, 1968, *203*, 79.

REGNAULT (F.). — *Ann. Oculist.* (Paris), 1973, *206*, 885.

REGNAULT (F.), BONSCH (N.), PASTICIER (M.), KERN (P.) and ROMQUI« (N.). — *Bull. Soc. franç. Ophtal.*, 1972, *85*, 221.

REGNAULT (F.), CASTANY (M. A.) and BRÉGEAT (P.). — *Presse méd.*, 1970, *78*, 1155.

REGNAULT (F.), DURAND (M.), KERN (P.) and LAURENT (M.). — *Bull. Soc. Ophthal. Fr.*, 1973, *73*, 519.

REGNAULT (F.), PASSA (Ph.), BABINET (J. P.) and CANIVET (J.). — *Bull. Soc. franc. Ophtal.*, 1970, *83*, 268.

RIASKOFF (S.). — *Die diabetische Retinopathie und ihre Behandlung mit Lichtkoagulation.* 'S-Gravenhage, Junk, 1972, 161.

RICCI (A.). — *Mod. Probl. Ophthal.*, 1972, *10*, 545.

ROOT (H. F.). — *Diabetes*, 1955, *4*, 386.

ROOT (H. F.). — *Med. clin. N. Amer.*, 1965, *49*, 1147.

ROOT (H. F.), MIRSKY (S.) and DITZEL (J.). — *J. Amer. med. Ass.*, 1959, *169*, 903.

ROTH (J. A.). — *Brit. J. Ophthal.*, 1969, *53*, 16.

ROULIER (A.). — *Graefes Arch. klin. exp. Ophthal.*, 1971, *181*, 281.

RUBINSTEIN (K.) and MYSKA (V.). — *Brit. J. Ophthal.*, 1972, *56*, 1.

SCHIFFER (H. P.) and BONNET (M.). — *Klin. Mbl. Augenheilk.*, 1974, *165*, 704.

SCHLESINGER (F. G.), FRANKEN (S.), VAN LANGE (L. T. P.) and SCHWARZ (F.). — *Acta med. scand.*, 1960, *168*, 483.

SCHÖFFLING (K.) and GRAEVE (R.). — *Med. Welt*, 1956, *25*, 627.

SCHOTT (K.). — *Ber. dtsch. ophthal. Ges.*, 1964, *66*, 349.

SCOTT (G. I.). — *Proc. roy. Soc. Med.*, 1951, *44*, 743.

SCOTT (G. I.). — *Brit. J. Ophthal.*, 1953, *37*, 705.

SCOTT (J. D.). — *Mod. Probl. Ophthal.*, 1969, *8*, 505.

SCOTT (J. D.). — *Mod. Probl. Ophthal.*, 1972, *10*, 680.

SCOTT (J. D.). — *Trans. ophthal. Soc. U.K.*, 1973, *93*, 373.

SÉVIN (R.). — *Fortschr. Augenheilk.*, 1971, *24*, 315.

SÉVIN (R.). — *Ophthalmologica* (Basel), 1972*a*, *165*, 71.

SÉVIN (R.). — *Bull. Soc. franç. Ophtal.*, 1972*b*, *85*, 213.

SÉVIN (R.) and CUENDET (J. F.). — *Bull. Soc. franç. Ophtal.*, 1969*a*, *82*, 170.

SÉVIN (R.) and CUENDET (J. F.). — *Ophthalmologica* (Basel), 1969 *b*, *159*, 126.

SÉVIN (R.) and CUENDET (J. F.). — *Ophthalmologica* (Basel), 1971, *162*, 33.

SHAFER (D. M.) — *Mod. Probl. Ophthal.*, 1972, *10*, 677.

SHEA (M.). — *Canad. J. Ophthal.*, 1972, *7*, 268.

SIMONSEN (S. E.). — *Congr. XXI Ophthal. septentr.*, 1973. *Acta ophthal.* (Kbh.), 1974. Suppl. 123, 223.

SINGH (P.), McDEVITT (D. G.), McKAY (J.) and HADDEN (D. R.). — *Hormone Res.*, 1973, *4*, 293.

SIPERSTEIN (M. D.), UNGER (R. N.) and MADISON (L. L..) — *J. clin. Invest.*, 1973, *47*, 1968.

SORSBY (A.). — The incidence and causes of blindness in England and Wales 1948-1962. *Rep. Pbl. Hlth & Med. Subj.* No. 114, London, H.M.S.O., 1966.

SPALTER (H. F.). — *Amer. J. Ophthal.*, 1971, *71*, 242.

SPALTER (H. F.). — Diabetic retinopathy: problems and management, *in* BELLOWS (J. G.) (Ed.): *Contemporary Ophthalmology.* Baltimore, Williams and Wilkins, 1972, 325.

TAKAKU (I.), KIRISAWA (N.) and CHIBA (M.). — *Atherogenesis.* Amsterdam, Excerpta Medica, International Congress Series no. 201, 1969, 189.

TASMAN (W.). — *Mod. Probl. Ophthal.*, 1972, *10*, 319.

TAYLOR (E.). — *Brit. J. Ophthal.*, 1970, *54*, 535.

TAYLOR (E.) and DOBREE (J. H.). — *Brit. J. Ophthal.*, 1970, *54*, 11.

TICHO (U.) and PATZ (A.). — *Amer. J. Ophthal.*, 1973, *76*, 880.

URRETS-ZAVALÍA (A.). — *Le Décollement de la Rétine.* Paris, Masson, 1968, 567.

URRETS-ZAVALÍA (A.). — *Bull. Soc. franç. Ophtal.*, 1973, *86*, 306.

URRETS-ZAVALÍA (A.). — Treatment of diabetic retinopathy. *Acta XXI Conc. ophthal.* (Gallia), 1974, *To be published.*

VALDORF-HANSEN (F.), HOYER (I.) and LARSEN (N. W.). — *Acta ophthal.* (Kbh.), 1969, *43*, 414.

VAN ECK (W. F.). — *Amer. J. Med.*, 1959, *27*, 196.

VAN HEUVEN (W. A. J.). — *Mod. Probl. Ophthal.*, 1972, *10*, 684.

VASCO-POSADA (J.). — *XXI Conc. Ophthal. Acta.* Mexico, 1970, *2*, 1561.

VASCO-POSADA (J.). — *Ann. Ophthal.*, 1972, *4*, 48.

VERHOEFF (F. H.). — *Trans. Amer. ophthal. Soc.*, 1947, *45*, 194.

VINK (R.) and NIEUWENHUIS-KOSTER (B. H. C.). — *Ophthalmologica* (Basel), 1973, *167*, 440.

WAITE (J. H.) and BEETHAM (W. P.). — *New Engl. J. Med.*, 1935, *212*, 367.

WESSING (A.). — *Klin. Mbl. Augenheilk.*, 1972, *160*, 274.

WESSING (A.) and BÖCKENHOFF (I.). — *Klin. Mbl. Augenheilk.*, 1951, *158*, 212.

WESSING (A.) and VOGEL (M.). — Xenon arc therapy or diabetic retinopathy, *in* FRANÇOIS (J.) (Ed.): *Symposium on Light Coagulation.* The Hague, Junk, 1973, 71.

WETZIG (P. C.). — *Mod. Probl. Ophthal.*, 1972, *10*, 350.

WETZIG (P. C.) and JEPSON (C. N.). — *Amer J. Ophthal.*, 1966, *62*, 459.

WETZIG (P. C.) and JEPSON (C. N.). — *Trans Amer. Acad. Ophthal.*, 1968, *71*, 902.

WETZIG (P. C.) and WORLTON (J. T.). — *Brit. J. Ophthal.*, 1963, *47*, 539.

WHITE (P.). — *Diabetes*, 1960, *9*, 345.

WHITE (P.). — *Med. Clin. N. Amer.*, 1965, *49*, 1015.

WHITE (P.), GILLESPIE (L.) and SEXTON (L.). — *Amer. J. Obst. Gyn.*, 1956, *71*, 57.

WHITE (P.) and YASKOW (E.). — Sth. med. (Bgham, Ala), 1948, *41*, 561.

WILLIAMSON (J. R.), VOGLER (N. J.) and KILO (C.). — *Med. Clin. N. Amer.*, 1971, *55*, 847.

WISE (G. N.). — *Trans. Amer. ophthal. Soc.*, 1956, *54*, 729.

WISE (G. N.), DOLLERY (C. T.) and HENKIND (P.). — *The Retinal Circulation.* New York, Harper & Row, 1971, 421.

WOLTER (J. R.). — *Acta ophthal.* (Kbh.), 1964, *42*, 971.

WOLTER (J. R.) and KNOBLICH (R. R.). — *Brit. J. Ophthal.*, 1965, *49*, 246.

WRIGHT (A. D.), KOHNER (E. M.), OAKLEY (N. W.), FRASER (T. R.), JOPLIN (G. F.) and HARTOG (M.). — *Brit. med. J.*, 1969, *2*, 346.

YALOW (R. S.) and BERSON (S. A.). — Radioimmunoassay of human growth hormone in plasma: principles, practices and techniques, *in* PECILE (A.) and MÜLLER, (E. E.) (Eds.): *Growth Hormone.* Amsterdam, Excerpta Medica Foundation, 1968, 60.

YANKO (L.), TICHO (U.) and IVRY (M.). — *Acta opththal.* (Kbh.). 1972, *50,* 556.

YANKO (L.), UNGAR (H.) and MICHAELSON (I. C.). — *Acta ophthal.* (Kbh.), 1974, *52,* 150.

YODAIKEN (R.) and DAVIS (E.). — *Diabetes,* 1974, *23,* 386.

YOUNG (F. G.). — *Lancet,* 1937, *2,* 372.

ZETTERSTROM (B.). — *Acta ophthal.* (Kbh.), 1972, *50,* 351.

ZWENG (H. C.). — Verbal communication, 1973.

ZWENG (H. C.), LITTLE (H. L.) and HAMMOND (A. H.). — *Trans. Amer. Acad. Ophthal.,* 1974, *78,* 195.

ZWENG (H. C.), LITTLE (H. L.) and PEABODY (R. R.). — *Laser Photocoagulation and Retinal Angiography.* Saint Louis, Mosby, 1969, 136.

ZWENG (H. C.), LITTLE (H. L.) and PEABODY (R. R.). — *Arch. Ophthal.,* 1971, *86,* 395.

ZWENG (H. C.), LITTLE (H. L.) and PEABODY (R. R.). — *Trans. Amer. Acad. Ophthal.,* 1972, *76,* 990.

INDEX

Masson

120, boul. Saint-Germain, Paris (VIe)

Dépôt légal : 1er trimestre 1977

Imprimé en France

Imprimerie l'Union Typographique
Villeneuve-Saint-Georges (V.-de-M.)

No d'impression : 525E 76